What's in This Book . . .

Dr. Bernard Jensen speaks from more than fifty years of research and practice. He offers common-sense answers to important questions now faced by the healing arts community—a community that includes the fields of iridology, homeopathy, chiropractic, acupuncture, and osteopathy. His years of experience have given him a wisdom that is unique in this age of instant cures and vascillating opinion. Dr. Jensen's ideas are practical; at the same time, they may be the catalyst for further exploration and discovery.

The practitioner of the natural healing arts realizes that this is a time when many live on a diet of colas, fast food, and sugar-laden desserts. In contrast, Dr. Jensen espouses a lifestyle that is natural, whole, and pure. And, he explains how health practitioners can work together to make their patients achieve optimum health. His down-to-earth advice makes too much sense to be overlooked. Anyone who knows the value of natural healing will find that the ideas within are essential to the future of the natural healing arts.

Dr. Bernard Jensen

BEYOND BASIC HEALTH

BERNARD JENSEN, D.C., Ph.D.

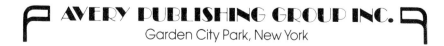
AVERY PUBLISHING GROUP INC.
Garden City Park, New York

The medical and health procedures in this book are based on the training, personal experiences, and research of the authors. Because each person and situation is unique, the editor and publisher urge the reader to check with a qualified health professional before using any procedure where there is any question as to its appropriateness.

The publisher does not advocate the use of any particular diet and exercise program, but believes the information presented in this book should be available to the public. If you have a history of back troubles, or other physical restrictions, we recommend that you consult with your health care provider before beginning any exercise program.

Because there is always some risk involved, the author and publisher are not responsible for any adverse effects or consequences resulting from the use of the suggestions, preparations, or procedures in this book. Please do not use the book if you are unwilling to assume the risk. Feel free to consult a physician or other qualified health professional. It is a sign of wisdom, not cowardice, to seek a second or third opinion.

Cover design by: Martin Hochberg and Rudy Shur
In-house editor: Karen Price Heffernan
Typesetting: Comart Graphics, Inc.

Library of Congress Cataloging-in-Publication Data

Jensen, Bernard, 1908-
    Beyond basic health.

    Includes index.
    1. Iris (Eye)--Examination. 2. Nutrition.
3. Diet therapy. I. Title.
RC73.5.J46 1988   616.07'545   88-26274
ISBN 0-89529-404-4

Copyright © 1988 by Bernard Jensen

Printed in the United States of America

10 9 8 7 6 5 4 3 2 1

Contents

PART ONE: THE IMPORTANCE OF IRIDOLOGY

When iridology is practiced in conjunction with nutrition, optimum health can be achieved. Iris analysis is used to spot the areas of weakness in the body, and nutrition is used to replace the damaged tissue in these areas with tissue that is new and healthy.

A language for iridology must be developed so that the terminology of Western medicine is no longer used by those in the natural healing arts. This language should be based on the basic iridology concepts: inherent weakness, chemical deficiencies, toxic settlements, tissue underactivity/overactivity, and tissue integrity.

The iris acts as a window to the body. In the future, the iridologist will be able to work with others in the natural healing arts to evaluate the effectiveness of other treatments. Iridology will also help people as they attempt to become healthier and stronger so that their children will not inherit their physical weaknesses.

There are so many things that iridology can reveal: it can locate inflammation, determine tissue integrity, locate toxic material and mineral deficiencies, monitor the health of the elimination channels, and many other things. This chapter details the uses—and limits—of the art of iris analysis.

The new-day doctor should not wait for people to become ill before he treats them; he should practice preventive health care and should be aware of the ways that diet and environmental conditions affect humanity. The patient must also do his part, and cooperate with the doctor.

PART TWO: THE CONSEQUENCES OF AN UNNATURAL LIFESTYLE

It would be ideal if we were all put on the pathway to health at the time of our birth. However, few people raise their children to follow "nature cure principles"; the choice to follow the path of natural health is one most of us face as adults. If we choose this path, we can be sure that we will reap rewards; if we stay on the pathway to disease, we will suffer the consequences.

Today, many illnesses are caused by the treatment of symptoms with suppressive drugs. These symptoms should instead be treated as manifestations of chemical deficiencies, and treated through diet. Food will be the medicine of the future.

Miasms are toxic accumulations that are often the result of the long-term use of drugs. Chemicals from drugs taken by our ancestors are passed down through generations. Chemicals also are ingested when we eat, drink, and breathe. Alleviation of this toxic-laden condition is a long-term process.

All drug residues should be eliminated from the body, and iridology should be implemented during the elimination process to monitor the patient's progress. Iridology can identify drug deposits, and reveal when they are gone.

Dr. Jensen believes that both Herpes II and AIDS are the result of the use of drugs for the suppression of other sexually transmitted diseases. This has caused the venereal taint to be driven deeper and become more highly concentrated. Instead of suppressing these diseases, their *causes* should be dealt with.

PART THREE: BUILDING HEALTH NATURALLY

biochemical salts. Dr. Jensen also uses natural foods in place of cell salts, with excellent results.

No one has a body that is working at 100 percent of its potential. The iridologist is most effective in ensuring that good health comes to the patient. He does this through cleansing the body, determining which nutrients the organs need, and restoring the brain and nervous system.

To Dr. Donald Bodeen and his wife, Joyce, staunch friends who are following the light of the full meaning of healing for mankind.

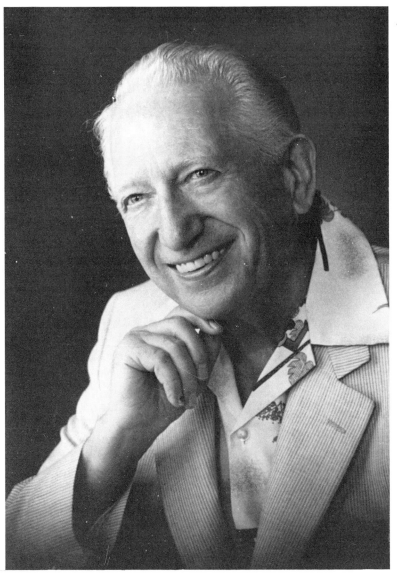

Dr. Bernard Jensen

Introduction

MAN'S IMMORALITY TO MAN

My teacher, Dr. V.G. Rocine, once said that a normal man is a moral man. He believed it was his moral obligation to teach man a healthy way of life. He said that the knowledge of nutritionally important chemicals and the curative diet is important for every man and woman who has anything to do with curing, teaching, hiring, directing, or advising people. Food science, Dr. Rocine said, should be taught in schools, colleges, and universities until every person knows how to avoid a disease-producing diet and knows what is, for him, a curative diet.

Hippocrates had the same idea. Hippocrates said we will never understand disease until we know our foods. He didn't have a knowledge of the chemical elements in foods, but he knew foods well enough to use them to treat certain ailments in the body. He also advised his patients on right-living habits.

Legislation against crime, drugs, and vicious habits is useless as long as man continues abnormal health practices. A normal person does not steal, murder, or commit outrages. We cannot legislate calcium into the bones, iron into the blood, sodium into the secretions, or potassium into the muscles any more than we can legislate bloom into faded cheeks or strength into our muscles. Education, however, can accomplish these ends.

This is not simply a health issue. It is a moral issue. Lack of teaching on the subject of health is a sign of man's immorality to man.

Good health enables doctors to cure, teachers to teach, moralists to moralize, ministers to save souls, and businessmen to succeed. Health enthusiasts, athletic instructors, school superintendents, teachers, psychiatrists, criminologists, jailers, judges, and anyone else who works with people can never fully understand man and his needs nor formulate practical systems for treatment, training, hiring assistance, and so forth until they have an intimate knowledge of the effects of nutrition on people and their behavior. They need to know how people act, what their mental faculties are and, especially, how to find out what chemical deficiencies may be related to occupational diseases and constitutional symptoms and characteristics. They also need to know how drugs, climates, poisons, and food additives affect each type of person. If crime is immoral, it is even more immoral to keep the criminal enslaved to his crime by not teaching him proper diet and health habits.

It is not enough to know about proteins, carbohydrates, fats, and calories. We must also know about the chemicals, minerals, and salts that are necessary for functioning of the blood, organs, secretions, tissues, and for health in general. We should also know which substances may be detrimental to human health: acids, poisons, and adulterants in manufactured foods, drinks, beverages, and over-the-counter drugs.

CONSUMER RIGHTS MUST BE GUARDED

To guard our health, every food and drug manufacturer should be under the strict surveillance of a chemist who can represent the welfare of the people. This chemist should have the legal power to forbid the use of harmful adulterants and preservatives in foods, drinks, tonics, and powders. He should positively forbid the manufacturer to rob food of its most essential nutrients.

It is essential that we have doctors and chemists who can advise us of the detrimental effects, side effects, hormonal effects, and brain effects of the drugs we have to use. We should be aware that drugs affect every aspect of our physical and emotional state. Drugs even affect our sex lives.

Our health must also be guarded by those who plant and tend the soil. Every farmer should study his soil to learn its chemical composition and what special plants, seeds, fruit trees, and berry bushes are best for scientific food production in that particular soil and climate. The farmer should know even more than the agricultural chemist. He should know about the organic sheet method of composting and how to replace soil with the nutrients it loses after harvest.

The earth has been greatly changed since man prostituted it and depleted its nutrients. Man's immorality to man continues as each generation leaves the next generation a planet that is more polluted and less fit to live in.

COOKING AS CHEMISTRY

People should be taught how to cook to meet the needs of individuals. It is criminal how people are released from the hospital after an operation without being taught how to change their lifestyles for the better. People should be taught how to positively alter their diets. They should be taught how to cook nutritious foods, how long to cook them, and what kinds of vessels to cook them in. They should be given a practical course in food chemistry that they can take home and use in their own kitchens.

The cook should know how to prepare foods without wasting the most valuable elements, and should understand the differing dietary needs of people. Since the cook's husband or wife or children may be different from the cook, they may have to be fed differently. The cook must be taught the physical and mental needs of those who eat her preparations. She should know how to cook for people of different ages, what foods are beneficial in summer, and what changes in diet are important during winter months. She should know how to cook for people who have neurotic habits, drinking tendencies, or criminal leanings. Until those who prepare food are taught the chemistry of food, sickness will continue to be a way of life.

OXYGENATION AND PURIFICATION

Oxygen is important for every organ in the body. When we have the proper amount of oxygen, we have strength and vigor. We can work longer and play harder. People need to know about oxygenation.

To purify blood for internal and external oxygenation, it is advisable to have fresh air day and night. We should also spend much time in the sunshine, breathe fresh air in abundance, and, if necessary for health reasons, live at a high altitude where the sky is blue, the air is breezy, and oxygen is present in abundance. It is also imperative to use foods that contain chemical salts needed by the blood and tissue. When these salts are adequate, we may obtain enough oxygen whether we work out at a fitness center or not.

If we have iron in our blood and potassium salts in our tissues, the circulating blood in the lungs absorbs oxygen and carries it to all the tissues in the body. The blood becomes pure: the body gains vigor, the cheeks gain blood, there is a stir in the arteries, strength in the muscles, recollection in the memory, and quickening in the intellect.

On the other hand, when iron and potassium are lacking and oxidation is low, the blood becomes impure and the circulation sluggish. Low oxygenation results in rapidity and weakness of the pulse, low vitality, and nervousness. The lean become leaner, the obese grow larger, and more catarrh, tonsillitis, muscular fatigue, sleepiness, rheumatism, neuritis, gout, acidity, and other ailments result from defective oxygenation.

The secretary who lacks oxygenation sits on her chair and becomes so nervous that she feels like jumping out of her skin and is, in her own words, "going to pieces." She is dizzy, hears noises, and her limbs go to sleep. She is excitable, irritable, hard to please, and easily fatigued, mentally and physically. Doctors are inclined to blame her work habits, or they say that the air in the office building is polluted, or that her apartment is overheated. However, the trouble is not in the air or with her work, her rooms, or the factory. It is her diet that is the cause. She needs, as we all do, adequate iron salts and potassium in her diet. Proper nutrition will provide this. People should be taught about oxygenation, because so many suffer from low energy and exhaustion.

POSITIVE THINKING MEANS GOOD HEALTH

Those who study mental states and their effect upon secretions, the blood, and the lymph, will soon learn how various emotions, passions, and unfavorable states of mind affect the chemistry of the entire body. It is important for anyone who wishes to enjoy perfect health to concentrate on feelings of love and optimism so that those chemical elements and salts that are needed for perfect metabolism will be secreted.

A positive state of mind is essential because it helps optimize the body's assimilation and metabolism of oxygen with the assistance of iron and potassium salts. This state of mind also fosters a greater degree of life, pleasure, vitality, and prosperity.

Until we realize that we have a moral obligation to teach people about nutrition and food chemistry, we are never going to have the bodily changes, tissue changes, and organ changes that are necessary to have a body in full health. There are so many things that are working against this moral obligation that we will have to resort to a strict, radical method to make the proper changes.

HOW I CAME TO THESE CONCLUSIONS

Over a period of years I have studied to see how man can improve his healing activities. During these years I have seen so many people get well after I advised appropriate changes in diet, exercise, and lifestyle.

I remember one time my wife and I were in an elevator in Sacramento, and a woman standing next to us said, "You're Dr. Jensen, aren't you?" I said "Yes." And she said, "Nineteen years ago I came to you in a wheelchair, with multiple sclerosis, and today I am free of it. There are no signs of it whatsoever. I have you to thank for that."

Another time, I was in a little Mexican cafe, and a lady recognized me and approached me. She said, "I want to thank you for what you have done for my arthritis. I have used alfalfa tablets continually for many years, and I am free of arthritis now."

I wish I could tell you all the stories that I have heard over the past years. I wish you could see the testimonials that have come to my office, describing how lives have been changed. These people changed their lives by stepping on to the path of right living, and they found that their new life was better than they had ever hoped it would be. Below, some of the areas I studied that led me to these conclusions are discussed.

The Influence of Hippocrates

One of my greatest inspirations has been Hippocrates. Hippocrates was a man dedicated to helping people with diseases and ailments. He lived in the fourth century B.C. on the island of Cos, one of the Greek islands.

Hippocrates cured people with food. People came from all over to see him. He taught his students how to use food to take care of people, and showed them that different foods have different effects on the body. Hippocrates described how he worked with the humors in the body, with the phlegm in the body, and with the wind in the body. Hippocrates reasoned that people had problems because of how they were living and what they were eating. He saw these problems leave when he changed the food habits of these people.

The Hippocratic Oath, used by medical doctors in the West, is very famous. He tried to influence the ethics of ancient doctors by giving them the proper principles to start with. I have often said that if we have men who are dedicated from the heart out, then we find that the healing art is secure in the hands of such persons. You will find that they are seekers. They want to know and do the right thing.

Hippocrates taught that sickness is a result of the type of life we live or the food we eat. If things aren't right, our bodies will tell us that it is time for a change.

Hippocrates made changes in diet and many people got well. One very important principle that I learned from Hippocrates is this: we will never understand disease until we know our foods.

V.G. Rocine

I learned more about this from V.G. Rocine, a Norwegian homeopath who had studied the work of the pioneering European food chemists and had brought this information to the United States. It was exciting to hear Rocine lecture about the chemical salts in food. He often compared the chemical salts in fruit and vegetables to the chemical salts used in homeopathic remedies.

Like Hippocrates over 2,000 years before, V.G. Rocine taught that food should be our medicine. He believed that nature had designed particular food types to contain chemical salts and other important nutrients in exactly the right concentrations and combinations to maintain a healthy chemical balance in the human body. He was among the first in the health arts to understand the importance of accurate quantitative analysis of the chemical composition of the ash left when food substances were burned up under controlled laboratory conditions. Once the amount of each chemical salt in each food was known, we could begin to use food to meet chemical deficiencies associated with diseases and other abnormal health conditions. We could use food to restore health.

Dr. Rocine found that all food could be burned down into an ash and that ash has certain percentages of chemicals such as potassium, sodium, and phosphorus. He likened these food chemicals to the dust of the earth. Dr. Rocine showed me that every chemical element in the earth has its own characteristics and has its own story to tell, and he taught me those stories.

I began to understand how these chemical elements work in the body. I learned that silicon is the magnetic element in the body and that the nerve force does not work well in the body unless it has the proper amount of silicon. It was easier to see that the body needed vitamin B because of serious deficiency diseases like beriberi. However, I found out that without the proper chemical elements, vitamin B doesn't remain in the body. It needs silicon to work with.

Silicon is found in the slick surface coatings of grains, sprouts, and vegetables. There are ways of getting that silicon, to replace the amount used up in the body due to nerve-wracking work, anxieties, worry, and fretting. Mental attitude can determine the rate of use of certain chemical elements, and we need certain kinds of foods to replace those lost.

I would say that Rocine was a modern-day scientist. His finest work was to bring European food chemistry to America, and to help us understand it. Unfortunately, he wasn't appreciated, and he didn't have the ability to promote his own work. I spent many years studying with him, and the most important thing he taught me was that healing comes from having the proper chemical balance in the body. The proper chemical balance is primarily determined by diet.

Some of those chemicals that balance the body are calcium, which is called the "knitter" in the body, and sodium, the "youth element." Sodium keeps us young and active, youthful, limber, and pliable. I began to see the need for these elements when my patients were complaining of certain symptoms. I could see these symptoms were due to a lack of certain chemical elements. When I added foods rich in these elements to their diets, the symptoms of disease went away.

This realization brought the first big change in my work. It showed me that the foods we eat have an effect on disease and ailments in the body, and that every disease, every ailment, and every sickness is accompanied by a lack of certain chemical elements. More than anything else, restoring balance to the chemistry in our body is the one thing that brings my patients back to health. I teach my patients that they must have this chemical balance to stay well.

At my ranch, I taught thousands of people how to get well and stay well, showing them how to use whole, pure, natural foods. I taught them that they had better learn how to take care of their bodies or doctors would make a living on their wrong living habits. If they wanted to have happy, healthy, prosperous lives, then they must be wholly well.

Ignatz Von Peczely—The Founder of Iridology

In my study of iridology, I was most influenced by Ignatz Von Peczely, the founder of iridology. Von Peczely had an unusual experience with an owl. At the age of eleven, he was trying to free the owl from his parents' garden when it clawed him and he accidentally broke its leg. He then noticed the appearance of a little brownish mark in the owl's eye. That mark later became a dark brown circle.

At first, I didn't believe this story. It is very hard to believe that a boy would notice a small mark in an owl's eye. But the more I learned about Von Peczely, the more I came to believe the story.

While attending school in Hungary, young Ignatz was known for his keen powers of observation and artistic ability. He was able to make wood carvings of actual people that were so exact that they were recognizable—a rare talent for a child. His teachers wanted to send him to Rome for further training in carving, but his parents would not allow him to go.

Because of the unique genius of this lad, I believe that the owl incident not only happened, but that it made a profound impression on him. This is when he began to develop the elements of a new system of health analysis.

Some years later, Ignatz looked into a man's eyes and told him that he had trouble with one of his legs. The man said, "Yes—how did you know?" Von Peczely replied, "I once had an experience with an owl with a broken leg, and what I saw in his eye I now see in yours." This man became a wonderful patient and a good friend. Von Peczely went on to cure one patient after another.

Iridology was a very crude science to begin with. But Von Peczely was able to put it together, and I think he organized it very well, because of his gift for accuracy and precision. He started by making a kind of "map" of the organs, glands, and other parts of the body, showing exactly where they correspond to the iris.

Dr. Von Peczely received his Doctor of Medicine degree in 1867 in Vienna. He soon became attracted to the use of homeopathic treatments, which I have also studied. Samuel Christian Hahnemann, a contemporary of Von Peczely who had studied at Leipzig and Vienna, had just developed the science of homeopathy, and this science was gaining a rapid reputation for its effectiveness. Many doctors opposed homeopathy as a fraud, but the proof was in the pudding. No one could deny that the dilute solutions of cell salts developed by Hahnemann were curing disease.

I believe that Ignatz Von Peczely was naturally drawn to homeopathy, because finding certain conditions in the iris indicated the need for treatment of these conditions. Dr. Von Peczely was not aware of the value of foods in the treatment of symptoms, and Western medicine wasn't advanced at the time, so it receive little attention.

Because iridology often revealed inflammation in the early pre-symptom stage, homeopathy was an ideal method of treatment. It was possible even then to see whether a treatment was working by monitoring the progress in the iris over a period of time. In my opinion, Dr. Ignatz Von Peczely was one of the most renowned and successful physicians of his time because of his effective use of iridology as a diagnostic aid.

The Hahnemann Therapy of Homeopathy

Dr. Hahnemann found, through experiment, that the same medications that produced certain symptoms in a well person would relieve the same symptoms in a sick person. When Hahnemann took quinine, he developed fever and chills—as if he had malaria. Hahnemann knew that quinine was also a very effective medication for those who actually had malaria. So, Hahnemann came up with the principle of homeopathic cure: "Like cures like."

Amazingly, the power of a medication was discovered, by Hahnemann, to increase in proportion to its degree of dilution. Most homeopathic remedies are in extremely small doses, which eliminates the problem of side effects. Homeopaths believe that the electromagnetically "potentized" medication is attracted to the cells deficient in particular cell salts and, as salts from the medications are drawn into these cells, an acute reaction is stimulated to throw off toxic accumulations.

Homeopathy is wonderful, but unless it is used together with a balanced diet and healthful lifestyle, there will be more problems, more breakdowns. It is the way we live that moves us either in the direction of health or disease, and proper foods are part of the health direction. Homeopathy works best when it is used with correct diet.

Like Dr. Rocine, I believe homeopathic principles are already incorporated in our foods, in the sense that the chemical elements in foods are in the right proportions and are properly "potentized" by sunshine and photosynthesis. With a proper knowledge of the chemical elements in foods, we can use foods at the homeopath uses cell salts, to correct nutrient imbalances, alleviate symptoms, and restore health. The symptoms of disease disappear as their causes are removed.

The Use of Herbs

Iridology and homeopathy are not the only healing arts I considered in my research. I also studied a system in Chinese medicine that dates back to 3000 B.C. In this system, there was no attempt to name diseases. Treatments were based on symptoms. Fevers were evaluated as to whether they were local or general. The pulse was a major source of information, and the type of pulse had several variations. Herbs were prescribed to relieve symptoms and balance the body, correlated with the times of year. Chinese herbal medicine is still an available option in modern hospitals in the People's Republic of China.

Herbs are foods. They contain certain chemical elements, vitamins, enzymes, and even unique ingredients. They can be effective in treating a person and they take care of many symptoms in the body.

I have used the herb rauwolfia to treat high blood pressure. The seeds and leaves of the foxglove plant were used to treat heart activity by herbalists before doctors began using it as digitalis. Some herbs act specifically on single organs in the body, or at least, more on one part than another.

The Value of Acupuncture

Acupuncture, one of the Eastern healing arts, also treats symptoms by removing their causes. It doesn't treat disease, per se. It may be used on multiple symptoms, but it is still treating symptoms. Restoration of adequate energy flow and balancing the energy flow system removes the cause of many symptoms.

Acupuncture is a mechanical approach that can harmonize with the chemical approach. It all fits in the wholistic perspective. Acupuncture works best when a diet of proper foods is also prescribed. Chemical elements repair and rebuild tissue. Energy flow alone, without the chemical elements, will not produce a complete man or a whole man.

Acupuncture allows the spirit to flow properly in the body. This talk about the spirit has nothing to do with some abstract thing off in the ether. It has nothing to do with occultism or spiritual activity or religion. This "spirit" is a kind of energy found in the magnetic qualities, the attractive energy. It can be related to the alchemy of the body and to the electromagnetic nature of the nerve impulses.

Man is a vibrant, electrical being, and he is a physical being. Even the cell structure has to have the right chemical elements to produce the electrical energy needed to draw some nutrients through the cell wall and keep others out. The pulling and pushing of these chemical elements follows electromagnetic laws, and this process helps build a healthy man. Acupuncture deals with the nerve meridians of the body, where stimulation with needles can release the nerve force to take care of a specific symptom or set of symptoms.

Chiropractic

Chiropractic is a system of mechanical manipulation that releases nerve force and restores communication between the brain and the organs and tissue structures of the body. Every organ in the body depends upon the brain. D.D. Palmer, who founded modern chiropractic, many times gave adjustments to only one part of the spine, the atlas. In moving the atlas, he was able to restore activity to many of the organs in the body through the nerves that branch off from the spinal column.

It is very important for the spinal nerves that carry the brain messages to be open and free and to have no blocks, or subluxations. The body has to be mechanically balanced. It is said that chiropractic was an art that first emerged in 1895 when D.D. Palmer hit a janitor in the upper part of his back with a cloth-wrapped brick and restored the man's hearing after he'd been deaf for many years.

One time I gave an adjustment to a woman who had epilepsy, and she had no more trouble after that. I wish I could do it again. What happened? I'm not sure. Perhaps miracles are sometimes stimulated in the nervous system. The nervous system has to be free flowing, but it also must have nourishment so it can recuperate, rebuild, and get rid of toxic acids.

I have treated other cases of epilepsy that took over two years for a complete change to come about. One particular lady in Pasadena, California, used to average fifteen to twenty epileptic spells a day, and after I worked with her for two years to stimulate the free flow of blood circulation and nerve supply throughout her body, she no longer had any epileptic spells. Her treatment also included proper foods. It didn't happen in ten minutes or two minutes, but her cure was still a miracle, and it was one of those things that we see happen when the nerve supply and the blood supply are free flowing.

The Palmer College of Chiropractic was founded in 1898. D.D. Palmer defined chiropractic as "the science of adjusting by hand any and all luxations of the articular joints of the body; more especially, the articulations of the spinal column, for the purpose of freeing any and all impinged nerves which cause deranged functions."

Chiropractors belong to the drugless arts and believe that the nervous system harmonizes all body functions, including defenses against disease. When the nervous system is impaired by any kind of pressure or blockage, it can't perform properly, and resistance to disease is lowered. (Modern science has validated this claim by observing a relationship between lymphocytes of several kinds and nerve ends in the body.)

According to chiropractic, even a slight misalignment (subluxation) of a spinal vertebra can cause interference with the spinal cord and nerves. The job of the chiropractor is to restore full nerve function by manipulating the misplaced vertebra until it is properly adjusted. Once the bones are back in place, nature does the rest.

Chiropractors take care of lumbago, slipped discs, arthritis, hay fever, high blood pressure, and other disorders. Many chiropractors also use nutrition, heat therapy, and other treatments along with mechanical adjustments. Some chiropractors use iridology, and many more have expressed interest, recognizing the tremendous potential value of its use as a diagnostic aid.

Osteopathy

Osteopathy, another drugless approach I am familiar with, was originally developed by Andrew T. Still, who made his system public in 1874. Still taught that all diseases are due to abnormalities in or near joints, and his recommended treatment for every disease was to locate and take care of these abnormalities. Still believed that drugs were poisons, and he opposed their use, advocating instead mechanical manipulation of the joints. He called these joint disturbances "subluxations," and claimed that they blocked the immune system from responding to the situation. Diseases, he taught, were caused when acidosis in the afflicated joint irritated nerves that were connected to more distant organs, causing reflex symptoms far from the original site of injury.

Over the years, osteopathy began to adopt many of the diagnostic, therapeutic, and philosophical approaches of Western medicine, including drugs to treat diseases. The D.O. license granted to osteopaths allows them to perform the same range of professional medical and surgical practices as medical doctors. There are, however, still some osteopaths who follow the drugless approach of Andrew Still, which they have expanded to consider the wholistic perspective.

Most osteopaths are more aware of the value of balanced nutrition than those who practice conventional Western medicine. Because iridology shows when a particular therapy or program is working well or failing to work, it would greatly assist the wholistic-oriented osteopaths.

The Importance of a Healthy Colon

At John Harvey Kellogg's sanitarium in Battle Creek, Michigan, it was found that the average colon actually has 15 percent beneficial bacteria and 85 percent undesirable bacteria. A healthy colon should have the reverse—15 percent undesirable bacteria and 85 percent desirable bacteria. The best way to stimulate better bowel health is to work to increase the good bacteria, such as lactobacillus acidophilus, and the toxin-producing, gas-generating undesirable bacteria will automatically diminish.

Elie Metchnikoff was a Russian-born bacteriologist of the latter nineteenth and early twentieth centuries who became head of the Pasteur Institute in Paris. He taught that intestinal underactivity and the putrefaction of its contents shortened life and attracted disease. Metchnikoff studied the centenarians among the Bulgarians and found that most of them used fermented milk.

When Metchnikoff studied what was in fermented milk, he discovered the lactobacillus Bulgaricus, and later the lactobacillus acidophilus was found in yogurt. The former could not live long in the bowel, but the latter thrived and tended to crowd out the undesirable bacteria. Metchnikoff's wonderful work emphasized the importance of bowel health and cleanliness, and his discovery of the lactobacillus pointed the way toward better bowel health.

In this century, Dr. Denis Burkitt, an English surgeon, pointed out the need for a fiber-rich diet to help prevent bowel disease. His pioneering study of rural East Africans (as compared to persons who live in cities) conclusively proved that high-fiber diets hastened bowel transit time and reduced bowel disease.

The use of iridology is one of the most effective and convenient ways to monitor bowel health. The iridologist can tell in a minute, from examining the iris, whether more fiber-rich foods are needed to stimulate increased bowel activity.

Other Health Arts

I became acquainted with a man in Canada who was involved in foot therapy. I saw a pile of crutches fifteen feet high that had belonged to people who had come to see this man. He manipulated their feet—nothing else—and after his treatment they were able to walk without the aid of crutches. It was a wonderful thing to see how foot therapy began to develop.

Eunice Ingraham worked with foot reflexology, which is a type of foot massage. Reflexology stimulates the organs of the body to action and also relieves pain.

Then, I studied craniopathy. This deals with adjusting the sutures of the skull. Major Jarnette from Nebraska did some wonderful work with the cranium and sacroiliac. This work has been done for many, many years.

Dr. William Albrecht, the head of the school of agriculture at the University of Missouri, has done wonderful work from a chemical standpoint. He corroborated what Dr. Rocine stated: that the soil needed care. If the soil does not contain the proper chemical elements, Dr. Albrecht taught, plant life will suffer.

When animals are grazed on land with the proper soil balance, they will avoid grass grown on poor soil, even if it's easier to get. How do the animals know what's right and what isn't?

At the Bircher-Benner Clinic in Zurich, Switzerland, Ralph Benner helped people learn the vegetarian way of life, and introduced them to a new way of living. Their lives were not only changed, but many of them were cured. It was from Ralph Benner that I found out about the elimination diet, which is helpful in cleansing the body of toxins.

All of these people helped me see that there were many ways of treating a person. I began to think that there must be some way I could incorporate a wholistic approach to healing in my own work. I could see that there was an overall goal to reach for, so I began to bring together all the best ideas from each of the great contributors to the health arts in my generation and the generation before it. I began to see that none of them treated people for disease. Most treated people to remove the causes of the symptoms.

A patient doesn't come in and say, "I'm troubled with cirrhosis of the liver." No one comes in and says, "I have glomerulonephritis," or "I have Bright's disease." All of these conditions are symptomatic, and the person who knows the internal conditions of the body well enough can treat these symptoms, because he knows the cause of that trouble.

IRIDOLOGY

I took up the science of iridology some years ago, because through it we were able to see tissue changes associated with the causes of most diseases. The iridologist can see signs of abnormal tissue activity in the body in four stages: the acute, subacute, chronic, and degenerative stages. These stages of activity can be seen as they grow progressively worse—acute to subacute, subacute to chronic, chronic to degenerative—each stage darker in the iris than the one before. We can also see these conditions reverse, as we change our way of living for the better—degenerative to chronic, chronic to subacute, subacute to acute, and then normal.

In thousands of eye pictures I have taken, I have observed the changes in the irides corresponding to the changes in the peoples' living habits. The healing process involves bringing in new tissue in place of old in the patient. Then, a reflex activity shows up in the iris that reveals very definite changes in the body. This is one of the most wonderful tools I could have hoped for to monitor the effectiveness of dietary changes on my patients' health. For this I owe a great debt to Ignatz Von Peczely, the "father" of iridology.

Of course, there were others who were doing the same thing. Joseph Angerer and Dr. Josef Deck of Germany have made great contributions to iris analysis. There are several thousand iridologists in Germany and the rest of Europe. In Europe, iridology was a favorite science among homeopaths. They would look at the iris to see what system was affected, and would feed the patient protomorphogens, which are dried, powdered organ substances from animal sources. They were very successful in helping their patients. These people were able to get rid of their problems. After studying their success, I also began to use protomorphogens when the circumstances called for them. When the pancreas is malfunctioning, for example, a person may benefit from pancreatic protomorphogen.

Many opponents of iridology say that it is not organized into a system. They say iridology is just hypothetical analysis. There's no such thing, they say, as a science of iridology. I could not disagree more.

In the iris, we find the health history of the patient. We see hereditary conditions. We may see psoric taints (an iris discoloration indicating a genetically inherited tissue abnormality caused by internally or externally generated toxic substances). We may see indications of a family history of drugs, scrofula, syphilis, gonorrhea, malaria. From what we see, we can tell where drugs have left taints and possible defects in the body for generation after generation.

We can see, in examining the iris, that there may be serious defects in the immune system. When our defenses against disease begin to break down, we become vulnerable to any plague, and we invite conditions that may become very serious in the future. Our only guarantee of immunity is a strong, clean, chemically balanced body.

The iris changes constantly. The iris represents cell structure, and the cell structure in the eye reflexly alters as the cell structure changes in any organ in the body. I began to see that there was a relationship between the two. Signs of underactive tissue and other abnormalities are evident, as are healing signs.

I found that using certain foods as treatment brought on the healing signs. Tissue changes could be verified from the iris much more reliably than by any other reflex analysis.

I began to prefer iridology as a form of examination. As I used it with my patients, I began to find out what the real basis for health was. I discovered that any chemically-deficient organ could successively go through four levels of tissue deterioration. But, I also found that certain foods or herbs could help these organs. I found out the chemical elements that were deficient and changed the patient's diet to supply the elements needed, resulting in repair and rebuilding of tissue. There were specific foods that tended to be more supportive of particular organs than other foods.

I studied with J. Haskell Kritzer, who wrote *Iridiagnosis*. I studied with Dr. Frederick Collins in Orange, New Jersey, who made me draw five hundred eyes in color, with all the various conditions I could find in the eyes, before I could graduate. I spent three years working with R.M. McLain every Wednesday and Friday night. We would go over pictures of eyes, checking every symptom we could possibly bring out from the iris.

We could identify over 60 percent of the problems before the patient even told us what was wrong.

Through iridology we can see many conditions and early problems developing that are preclinical, not yet manifesting as symptoms. Yet, as the body grows cleaner and stronger, the healing crisis that develops in the patient brings back symptoms they may have originally had ten or twenty years before. I began to see that there was a system emerging.

Dr. Henry Lindlahr said, "Give me a healing crisis, and I will cure any disease." When treatment was begun and the healing crisis occurred, the symptoms of ailments that people had before would reappear. Through trial and error, I discovered that this healing crisis could only be hastened by using foods rich in the chemical elements needed to feed the deficient tissues. The reversal would produce healing signs not by non-nutritional treatments alone, but in conjunction with chemical elements from foods.

In other words, once we open up the nerve force of the body through mechanical means such as chiropractic, we need to supply the foods that produce new tissue in place of the old. Healing sings don't come by mechanical change; they come by proper feeding of the chemical elements.

Rocine said, "Give me the proper chemical elements for tissue change in the body, and I will cure practically any disease." Rocine didn't mean that food chemistry is the only way to restore health. But without good nutritional support, no true healing correction takes place. And, if we brought *all* wholistic healing methods to work on a patient, I believe a wonderful cure could take place.

During the healing crises I took care of, I could see that I was dealing with pathology. In the iris I saw evidence of tissue change, and you can't verify tissue integrity through x-rays or blood tests. Many times I could see future problems developing in the iris that could not be diagnosed by other methods. There was no laboratory test that could spot these preclinical problems that were developing in the early stages of a disease, but the iris was able to reveal them.

After I gave a lecture at a college, one of the professors came up to me and said, "I'm glad I have the opportunity to meet you. Twenty-five years ago, you examined my father and mother. My father died of the problems you found by examining his iris. My mother is still alive, but she is having the problems you noticed in her eyes so long ago."

How is that possible? Is this a psychic business? Is this the product of an occult science? Iridology has a definite physical order and structure and is not just in the form of a hypotheses. Iridology is based on the research and experience of sincere and well-educated men, some of whom were ahead of their time (and possibly ours) in the quality of their thinking. How can scientists say iridology is only a hypothesis?

THE COMPUTERIZATION OF IRIDOLOGY

The computer is going to bring us to the next stage of advancement in iridology. The iridologist struggles to remember everything. He can't visually estimate anything smaller than about a tenth of an inch. A computer can measure down to twenty-five hundredths of an inch. That's the kind of accuracy we need. This is what we need to improve our analyses.

With the help of the computer, we will be able to do things now that are going to standardize our work in iridology. We will have a system that will show where every organ is represented in the iris. The computer will be able to go to the area of the iris that represents an organ, and scan it to measure the stage of inflammation it is in. It will give us the percentage of each stage of inflammation in each organ of the body.

This will standardize iridology analysis, reduce human error, and increase the amount of useful information available to the health arts professional. I am not satisfied with iridology as it is now. It is too much of a subjective analysis, and we need the refinement, accuracy, precision, reliability, and repeatability that a computer can give us.

We need the computer for a storage place for our findings. We need something that can compare iris pictures before and after, this year to last year. With a computer, we can check to see that the course of therapy the doctor is using is right. We have to check up on the food program we use, we need to know if we are treating the patient correctly or not.

Taking care of a patient does not simply mean getting rid of a pain and hearing the person say, "I feel well again." This is not reasonable. We find out that nine out of every ten people walking around say they feel well, but studies show two out of ten have a chronic disease. We must use iridology and computers to check the condition of the tissue, and work toward greater prevention, earlier recognition of problems, and earlier and more wholistic treatment.

THE FUTURE OF IRIDOLOGY

There are great things that iridology can do in the future. We need to monitor the elimination channels more carefully. What is the health status of these elimination channels? How can we prevent diseases of the bowel, lungs and bronchials, kidneys, and skin?

We will be able to investigate and closely monitor the development of osteoporosis, which is in epidemic proportions among elderly women.

The effects of drugs on tissues can be researched with help of computerized iridology. Today there are thousands of drugs made from petrochemicals or coal tar. We can't tell them apart with direct visual observation of the iris, but maybe the computer can.

I believe computerized iridology can be integrated with a complete program of foods and supplements to go along with each iris analysis—foods, vitamins, minerals, herbs, protomorphogens, and other supplements.

Ultimately, we are working for complete wellness in the body. This is the goal we have to work for. There are standards for health and nutrition that need to be developed.

We have to consider the mechanical arts, the personality, and the kind of brain material we have to work with. We have to develop criteria for priorities to decide what organ is in need of the greatest care. We have to locate every organ that is sick, underfunctional, and a drag to other organs.

I hope that someday people can learn iridology from a combination of computer learning programs and video lessons. I'm sorry to say this is one thing that is yet to come. The best way to learn iridology is to actually see iris slides and correlate symptoms with the signs we see in the iris. However, it shouldn't be a matter of taking care of symptoms anymore. We can tell what organ is affected, what its dominant stage of inflammation is, and what percentage of each stage of inflammation is represented in each affected organ.

When fifteen organs are simultaneously affected, we can get all kinds of misleading symptoms. If the one organ causing the most trouble is identified and taken care of, it will usually erase many of the symptoms and simplify the whole situation. Through proper feeding and proper treatments, we can eliminate symptoms. But, to go still farther into the reversal process, we would be able to predict the healing crisis and what systems and organs would be most affected. This would enable people to develop a wellness program so that the elderly, the handicapped, and the infirm could live in much better health, and wouldn't have to look forward to a convalescent home the rest of their lives to just stay alive.

We owe it to the next generation to have doctors who are going to teach us how to do our part. Then, the future generation will be all that it has the potential to be.

PART ONE
The Importance of Iridology

CHAPTER 1

The Iridology-Nutrition Connection

To be most effective, the science of iridology must be practiced in conjunction with nutrition. Iridology is the most effective means we have of identifying and locating chemically deficient tissue in the body. Nutrition is the only means we have of supplying the chemical elements needed to restore integrity and balance to that tissue. Iridology and nutrition complement one another perfectly, and an understanding of how these two healing arts go together makes it possible to take care of many conditions that may be difficult or impossible to take care of otherwise.

I believe all chronic diseases are accompanied by deficiencies in the chemical elements. We know what elements particular tissues and organs need, so if there was a way to "look inside" the body and see which organs and tissues were lacking in certain elements, we would know exactly what to do and what to prescribe.

The iridologist knows that there is a way to "look inside" the body. Iridology reveals specific areas of inflammation and inherent weakness in the body by reflex signs shown in the iris. These signs show exactly what organs, glands, and tissues are involved.

INHERENT WEAKNESSES AND NUTRITION

Whenever we have an inherent weakness in the body, it shows up in the iris as a separation of the iris fibers. This separation of fibers shows a different tissue structure, a different genetic pattern in that part of the body. By analogy, the texture of that tissue is like the grain of soft wood or the loose weave of a gunny sack, and it cannot use or store the chemical elements as efficiently as other tissue. Inherently weak tissue assimilates nutrients more slowly, depletes easily, and does not eliminate its metabolic wastes as fast as normal tissue. For this reason, inherently weak organs can't keep up the rate of activity or take the abuse and overwork that other organs can. They "run out of gas" more easily and frequently, so to speak. This makes them more susceptible to disease than other tissue.

However, if they are properly cared for, these inherently weak areas can serve us well. Prevention of chemical depletion is the key. To assure adequate function, the nutritional density of a weak organ must be sustained at a high level. Foods rich in the chemical elements needed by every organ must be used, and we need to know two things: what chemical elements predominate in certain tissues and which foods supply them. (The chemical elements needed by certain parts of the body are listed in Table 1.1.) We also need to realize that a person with certain inherent weaknesses cannot take stress, overwork, fatigue, and late night activities like others can, nor can he carry resentment and resistance and get away with it. He must find and live a lifestyle that is balanced physically, mentally, and spiritually.

Obviously, if we know which body tissues and organs are inherently weak, we can start feeding the nutrients—the biochemical elements needed—before disease symptoms manifest. That is, we can prevent disease by restoring chemical balance in the body before any of the symptoms recognized by Western medicine even appear. Similarly, when disease is already present, we can identify the involved parts of the body by iridology analysis, consider what chemicals are needed in each part, and select an array of foods to build up the body and supply all those chemical deficiencies. There are approximately ninety areas of the iris that correspond to different organs, glands, tissues, and systems. We have hundreds of foods to choose from, plus juices, herbs, teas, broths, tonics, and supplements. In various combinations, these natural remedies are capable of producing over a thousand different remedial effects.

Using iridology, we identify the organs and tissues that are inherently weak. Using nutrition, we supply the chemical elements needed by those organs and tissues to overcome their deficiencies. An iridology analysis cannot identify specific diseases, but it can and does pinpoint inherently weak tissue locations that are actual or potential sites of disease. By building up those parts of the body through nutrition, disease is prevented or overcome.

EACH ORGAN AND TISSUE STRUCTURE IS UNIQUE

Each specific type of tissue in the body, whether of bone, muscle, gland, or organ, has a different balance of chemical elements and a unique structure suited to its purpose in the body. Altogether, they are designed to work in harmony, with the brain as the symphony conductor.

One chemical element usually plays a central role in the chemistry of each organ, and that particular element gives that organ its unique character, chemically speaking. In each case, many chemical elements take part in the metabolism of an organ, but one predominates. For example, iodine plays the predominant role in the metabolism of the thyroid gland, and its deficiency leads to goiter and disruption of all body functions de-

Table 1.1   Chemical Needs of the Body

Body Part or System	Chemical Needs
Adrenals	Zinc (trace)
Bones	Fluorine, calcium, phosphorus
Bowel	Magnesium
Brain	Phosphorus, manganese, sulphur
Circulation	Sulphur, silicon, oxygen
Digestive system	Chlorine, sodium, potassium
Hair	Silicon
Heart	Potassium
Kidneys	Chlorine
Liver	Sulphur, iron
Lungs	Oxygen, iron
Nails	Silicon
Nervous system	Phosphorus, manganese, sulphur
Pituitary gland	Bromine
Respiratory system	Oxygen, iron
Secretions	Potassium, chlorine
Skin	Sulphur, silicon, oxygen
Spleen	Fluorine, copper
Stomach	Chlorine, sodium
Teeth	Fluorine, calcium, phosphorus
Thyroid	Iodine
Tissues	Potassium, chlorine, sulphur

pendent upon normal thyroid function. Sodium and potassium are found in every cell of the body, but sodium is of primary importance in the gastrointestinal tract and potassium is of primary importance to the heart and muscle tissue.

The character of an organ or tissue depends largely on the characteristics of its predominant chemical element. Calcium tissue, as in bone, functions much more slowly than tissue in which potassium, sodium, or iodine predominate, and there is a reason for this. The chemical composition and metabolic rate of each organ establish a certain vibratory rate, greatly influenced by the vibratory rate of the predominant element.

The vibratory level and metabolic rate of each organ, gland, and tissue type are initially increased at the first stage of deficiency of the predominant chemical element, then decreased as the deficiency persists. This is signaled by signs in the iris of an acute, subacute, chronic, or degenerative condition in the body, each of which indicates a certain level of tissue inflammation. Ongoing deficiency of a predominant element leads to a shift in the chemical equilibrium, activity level, and function of an organ.

THE FOUR STAGES OF INFLAMMATION

When the iridologist encounters an inherent weakness in the iris, he looks to see if it is in the stage of acute, subacute, chronic, or degenerative inflammation. The acute or hyperactive stage is indicated by white, raised iris fibers. The subacute, chronic, and degenerative stages are shown by increasingly darker shades of gray. The degenerative stage may appear as a black lesion. All four levels are associated with stages of inflammation and cell damage, and all four represent deficiency in a particular chemical element.

In the acute stage, the hyperactive tissue uses up the nutrients supplied to it at a rapid rate, much like a starving man greedily wolfing down food. At this stage, the concept of sustaining maximum nutrient density is important. We can pour in foods containing the needed biochemical elements, and we need to do that, but it will take a certain amount of time—weeks or months—for that organ to slow down to a normal metabolic rate while chemical equilibrium is reestablished.

The subacute, chronic, and degenerative stages are increasingly hypoactive, representing a slowing of the metabolic rate and a lowering of the vibrational frequency. The organ, either from drastic short-term deficiency or gradual depletion over a long period of time, undergoes progressive deterioration in chemical composition. Its power to attract the chemicals it lacks is reduced. Again, we must take care of the deficiency, but we face a different kind of problem than in the acute stage. In the acute stage, the organ uses the biochemical element supplied to it, but extremely rapidly and inefficiently. In the subacute, chronic, and degenerative states, the organ is increasingly handicapped in its ability to assimilate the chemicals it needs. Maintaining high nutrient density for such an organ is still important, but we must realize it can only take a little at a time. As its normal chemical equilibrium is approached and its vibrational level increases, the organ will be able to assimilate faster.

SOURCES OF CHEMICAL DEPLETION

We usually think of nutrient deficiency in the body in terms of inadequate diet, and that is often true. However, there are other sources. Through overwork, we can build up fatigue acids in the body. Excessive mental work can deplete the brain, nerves, and glands. We can build up toxic states in the body, leading to chemical depletion, by simply neglecting to get enough fresh air, sunshine, and exercise.

We use up chemical elements as we direct energy into activities and relationships in our work, marriages, and friendships. Some jobs draw more on our energy than others. Some people draw more on our energy than others. In fact, I believe that specific relationships can deplete one specific biochemical and not others. If we are married to a certain type of person, for example, we could become depleted of sodium and develop stomach, digestive, and bowel problems as a result. Our work could be of a type that drains us of iodine or silicon.

V.G. Rocine believed that people are differentiated into twenty temperament types, based on a predominant influence of one particular biochemical in each person. Different temperament types need certain kinds of foods to function normally. When we are unable to express our gifts, talents, and abilities, or when we express ourselves in excess, we may develop deficiencies, according to this idea.

To repeat, deficiencies may not express as symptoms for quite some time, and the particular symptoms that will express cannot be accurately predicted from iris analysis. The same basic set of inflammations in the same organs and tissues may express in one person as arthritis, in another as bronchial asthma, and in a third as cancer. We are all unique, and the biochemical patterns that make us who we are make it impossible to predict the specific end result of long-term chemical deficiencies.

WHEN SYMPTOMS APPEAR

The appearance of symptoms marks the clinical stage of disease. When the skin becomes dry, we know something is wrong. When we have pain in the shoulder, we know something is wrong. Excessive bloating, gas, constipation, or diarrhea tell us that something is wrong. Symptoms are consequences of deficiencies, inflammation, and chemical imbalance in the body. The iridologist can see the causes of these events in the iris, in lesions in the iris fibers that appear white, gray, dark gray, or black. All disease is preceded or accompanied by catarrh.

Although there is a point of no return in tissue damage caused by severe long-term deficiencies and toxic buildup, it is surprising to see how the body responds to nutritional correction in most cases. By proper dieting, using soups, supplements, herbs, broths, and tonics to bring in the needed chemical elements, we work toward remission and the reversal process, our goal being the healing crisis. When organs and tissues are inherently weak and deficient in chemical elements, toxic wastes tend to gather in them. These are thrown off during the healing crisis.

HEALING INVOLVES THE WHOLE BODY

It is easy to draw the mistaken conclusion that once we have identified the sources of inflammation in the body, all we have to do is feed the body the right foods with the chemical elements needed to take care of the deficiencies, and the problem will disappear. This mistake is based on the assumption that only the depleted portions of the body are "sick" and the rest of the body is "well." I have never encountered a case in which there was a diseased kidney in a well body, or an arthritic shoulder in an otherwise well body. Everything in the body depends upon everything else to a greater or lesser degree.

If the stomach and bowel are short of sodium, we can be sure that the rest of the body is affected by that sodium deficiency. If the hair and skin lack silicon, we know very well that the nerves are affected. In the case of underactive organs, all processes in the body normally affected by that organ will be operating under par to some degree.

Because disease centered anywhere in the body has exerted some effect on every other organ, tissue, and cell, we must take care of the patient by strengthening the whole body. Certainly, we must use more of the foods containing elements found to be deficient in various organs. But, we should also feed and exercise the rest of the body. We may find a kidney problem, but unless we build up the thyroid as we deal with the kidney, the metabolism will never become strong enough to throw off the toxic accumulations in the kidney.

Without nutrition, iridology is only an analytic tool to help us find what is wrong in the body. Without nutrition we don't know what to do to right the wrong. Food, then, becomes our best medicine. Most of the health arts can only find part of what is out of balance in a person and are capable of restoring, at best, only that part. For many years, people have been treated through drugs, surgery, chiropractic, and other methods. None of these can take the place of proper nutrition. Nutrition is the superior science in restoring the body to health.

Suppression of symptoms through drugs is not true healing. Symptoms disappear temporarily only to return later, worse than before. Iridology shows that drug residues remain in inherently weak and underactive tissue, producing toxic side effects, possible genetic damage, and time-bomb effects.

As we chemically feed the body properly, it becomes cleaner. Its power, vital force, activity, and youth return. The intermediate state or goal may be freedom from pain, freedom from discharges, and better health. The long-range goals should be vital health, high-level well-being, and longer life.

HOW NUTRITION WORKS WITH OTHER DRUGLESS ARTS

Very little can be done by any of the healing arts to get rid of a chronic disease that is rooted in chemical deficiency if nutrition is not used. The application of nutrition is required for optimum results.

Chiropractic is a wonderful science, and it has helped many thousands of people. But, nearly all chiropractors encounter patients who can't hold a spinal adjustment, and this may indicate a chemical deficiency.

Psychiatry, which is rapidly becoming a drug-oriented art, can do little for a patient whose mind is imbalanced due to chemical imbalance in the body.

Acupuncture, massage, osteopathy, and all the healing arts are ineffective in coping with nutritionally based problems. We need to be objective, whatever our field, and always take care of the chemical deficiencies first.

Once the body is in right chemical balance, the patient can benefit from mechanical adjustment and other therapies to restore nerve supply, blood flow, and so forth.

HEALING TAKES TIME

As we have seen in our discussion, a shortage of any chemical element needed by the body produces chemical imbalances that eventually result in symptoms of disease. The harsh consequences of deficiency do not happen overnight, but over long periods of time, which makes them relatively subtle processes, invisible on a day-to-day basis.

If we inadvertently cut down on iron-containing foods because of a shift in our food patterns, no symptom occurs from missing our eight to ten milligrams of iron the first day, nor the next. We may go on for weeks before noticing that we are tiring more easily, finding it harder to get up in the morning, and lacking our usual energy. These symptoms, however, are so general and nonspecific that few physicians would guess what was wrong. And because they are so gradual, we seldom realize that we are going downhill. Yet, dripping water wears away rock in time, and chemical depletion is similar. What we don't eat affects our lives as profoundly as what we do eat.

It would be wonderful if we could say exactly how much of each chemical element should be taken by the "normal" person to prevent disease and maximize high-level well-being, but we are all too different to make assumptions about exact nutrient needs. The Recommended Daily Allowances by the Federal Food and Drug Administration is a useful guideline. ("Normal" is a concept that can be best interpreted as absence of debilitating symptoms.)

HEALTH IS A WAY OF LIFE

When I say nutrition deserves the highest priority in the healing arts, I must also point out that health is more than nutrition. Health is a way of life. We need to learn how to relax, slow down, and be kind to others—including ourselves. We need to clean old, negative thoughts out of the closets of the mind, and understand and love people more. We need to appreciate what is wonderful about life instead of dwelling on its seamier aspects. We must eat right—but we must also live right for correct nutrition to make sense in the context of life as a whole.

Each individual is unique, and this uniqueness is apparent in the iris, which shows that each person has a slightly different set of inherent weaknesses and strengths. Basically, this means that your nutritional needs are not the same as mine. The husband's nutritional needs are not the same as the wife's. We should find out what our bodies need and make sure we get the foods containing those chemical elements.

SOME SPECIFIC EXAMPLES OF FOOD AS TREATMENT

As we view the iris, we may detect an overactive or underactive thyroid. This points to a need for iodine foods (fish, dulse). We may find anemia and know the blood needs iron (liver, beets, greens, prickly nettle), and the body needs exercise to move the blood around. We might discover darkness in the stomach area inside the autonomic wreath or signs of too much or too little hydrochloric acid, which means sodium is needed (whey, celery, papaya, okra). These are the sorts of conditions we look for in iridology to reveal deficiencies and demonstrate the need for particular foods or herbs.

The skin is a silicon organ. Although the greatest amount of silicon is stored in the skin areas, it is also used and stored in the nerves, nails, hair, and other parts of the body. If we see a gray ring around the iris (scurf rim), we know the skin is short of silicon, and we also know that if the skin is depleted chemically, all other parts of the body that use silicon will be deficient, too. If any of the organs have a shortage of a chemical needed for proper function, toxic materials can settle in that weakened tissue, because they will settle most in a chemically depleted organ.

NUTRITION AND THE HEALING CRISIS

Nutrition and iridology work together in demonstrating the truth of Hering's Law of Cure: "All cure works from the head down, from the inside out, in reverse order as the symptoms first appeared." As we strengthen the body through nutrition, exercise, and a right way of living, the brain centers and the glandular and nerve functions controlled by them become more active in revitalizing all the body's systems, and healing begins to come "from the head down." The digestion and assimilation improve as we eat right and the bowel, along with other elimination organs and systems, is cleansed and restored. The result of this is a cleaner bloodstream. With the elimination of toxins and the rejuvenation of tissue "from the inside out," we are preparing for the healing crisis, which is the goal of all natural healing. Healing lines in the iris grow acutely white as the healing crisis arrives. The healing crisis is a dramatic, usually brief period (about three days) when the patient re-experiences old symptoms, "in reverse order as the symptoms first appeared."

BALANCING YOUR DIET

A healthy way of living is not just diet, because diets are one-sided and only necessary to reach a balance. A healthy lifestyle requires an all-around, well-balanced eating regimen. The best diet, over a period of a day, is two different fruits, at least four to six vegetables, one protein and one starch, with fruit or vegetable juices between meals. Eat at least two green leafy vegetables a day. 50 to 60 percent of the food you eat should be raw.

Below are eight food laws I have devised to help you design a balanced diet.

1. We need whole, pure, natural foods.
2. We need six vegetables, two fruits, one starch, and one protein daily.
3. Our foods should be 80 percent alkaline and 20 percent acid.
4. We need a variety of foods.
5. Sixty percent of our food should be raw.
6. Natures cures, but she must have the opportunity.
7. Avoid overeating in general, and avoid eating a few foods to excess (as a habit) in specific.
8. Avoid deficiencies in your food regimen.

When you have established a balanced daily eating regimen, you can add to and rearrange your intake according to your occupation, ailments, marriage, and the type of body you possess. If it has been determined you need calcium or potassium, this can be added by way of a supplement, herb, or tonic. Usually, some specific foods high in the element needed are added with or between meals. For instance, rice polishings and extra sprouts are given if a person is in need of silicon. To a child needing calcium, green kale and barley soup may be given.

With chemicals and foods, a patient can be fed back to health and kept there through a maintenance program. However, it will be almost impossible to get a patient well if you don't know his needs or the chemical elements.

Nature has given us hundreds of foods that contain healing elements for our health and well-being. We should study these foods and analyze and understand the natural healing properties they contain. Many hundreds of commercial foods and drinks become slow-acting poisons *by default*, lacking the necessary chemical elements for maintaining and rebuilding the cells and tissues of the body. Applying the laws of health leads to liveliness, suppleness, strength, youthful freshness, and charm even into advanced years.

A genuine food chemist and nutritionist knows that the proper foods cure in one way—by building up the blood and toning up the organs, nerve centers, brain centers, and the glandular system. To accomplish this, we should tap into the best foods the earth, sea, and sun have to offer. When the once-deficient food elements are again supplied in the proper balance, the body and organs take on new strength and the mind gains new creative power.

All of these normalizing changes back up good health and can be viewed in the iris. This is the invaluable link iridology has in correlation with nutrition. There is no method as practical as iridology in monitoring the tissue changes that take place in the transition from disease to health and well-being.

THE HEALTH STAIRCASE

The importance of correct nutrition is emphasized by Dr. Barnet Meltzer's "Health Staircase" (Fig. 1.1) which begins with malnourishment at the bottom step and ends with optimal nourishment at the top. The effects, on a scale of 0 to 100, are expressed in terms of health level. Dr. Meltzer has established five fundamental categories of health status:

1. Optimal Nourishment: Optimal Wellness
2. Suboptimal Nourishment: Partial Wellness
3. Mediocre Nourishment: Average Health
4. Poor Nourishment: Poor Health
5. Malnourishment: Symptomatic Disease

These categories correspond to the five levels of nutritional status presented in Figure 1.1.

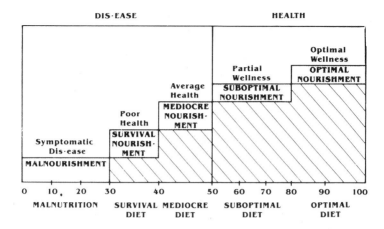

Figure 1.1   Dr. Meltzer's Health Staircase

Our goal, of course, would be to achieve optimal nourishment and optimal wellness. When this goal is achieved, the rewards that accompany right living will be ours. These rewards are:

- Real happiness
- Consistent sexual fulfillment
- Daily peace of mind
- Positive mental attitude
- No symptoms of illness
- Joyful sense of well-being, even in times of crisis
- Strong, physically-fit body

- Emotional fulfillment
- Proper body weight
- Joy of spiritual prosperity
- Emotional stability
- Meaningful relationships
- Balanced lifestyle
- Biochemical balance in the body

At the lower end of the health staircase, the chances are greatest for developing disease and disturbances of many possible kinds in the body—and in the mind. Notice on the scale of the chart that this is the lower 30 percent of the optimal level of wellness, a danger level. It is largely up to the individual to exercise responsibility over his or her nutrition, which means we ourselves determine our level of health.

Only foods and herbs can supply the right biochemicals to rejuvenate tissue damage by inflammation and disease. Drugs do not build new tissue. As the healing progresses and tissue is rejuvenated, iridology shows that white healing lines are coming into the dark lesions in the iris. This tells us the right foods with the right biochemicals are being used. Nature cures, repairs, rebuilds, and regenerates if we provide the right chemical elements. Iridology shows us what is wrong. Nutrition restores the balance, and iridology shows when healing is occurring. This is the iridology-nutrition connection.

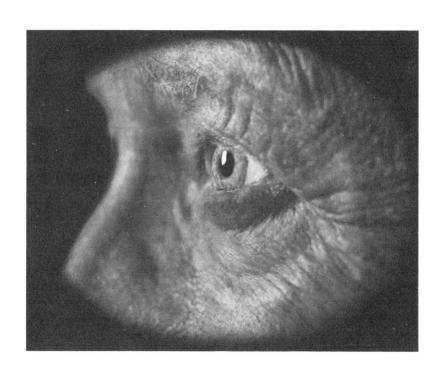

CHAPTER 2
Needed: A Language for Iridology

Modern iridology began in 1861 with the work of Dr. Ignatz von Peczely in Hungary. Now, the time has come where the need for a special language for iridology is evident.

In the past, iridology has borrowed its terms and concepts from Western medicine, homeopathy, naturopathy, and other disciplines—each of which has a tradition of its own language development. This borrowing has resulted in many misunderstandings. Too many iridologists use the language of Western medicine when they talk about diseases and treatments. Yet, iridology does not read "disease" in the eye.

There must be a language for the iridologist, through which we can talk about what we see in the iris and relate what we see very clearly and very objectively to the patient in terms of his or her health care needs. This language must be clear to the practitioner and clear to the patient. It must connect with our patients' complaints. It must be a language all drugless practitioners who use iridology can agree on.

Our patients, for the most part, come to us prepared to describe what is wrong in the language of Western medicine. "I have arthritis," a patient tells us, and we understand there is a joint inflammation in his body. "I have a cold . . . or I have the flu," another one says, and we know she is saying that she is going through a catarrhal elimination. The problem with this language difference is that disease or ailment names like arthritis, colds, flues, and diabetes, for example, have been developed from a tradition valuing a very mechanical view of the body and having a different approach to healing and treatment from the natural, drugless healing arts. For Western medicine, each disease or ailment represents a condition for which some "treatment of choice" is available. This treatment might include drugs, radiation, chemotherapy, or surgery. The goals of Western medicine practitioners sometimes include eliminating or suppressing the symptoms of disease, and sometimes include managing a chronic disease that is considered incurable, like arthritis. Their methods of prevention include vaccination. Often, the goal of Western medicine is to get a patient well enough to go back to work and to be able to function as a family member again.

Most of the natural, drugless healing arts will continue to use disease names, because they are convenient, but we need to change our language to distinguish our beliefs, values, and traditions from those of Western medicine. Our goal in health care, for example, involves a concept of correction of the problem, not just symptom relief. Our understanding of disease is that the same set of symptoms may develop in the body by many different pathways, which should be taken into consideration when we are deciding how to respond to our patient.

In the natural healing arts, we must always think in terms of treating the patient, not just the disease or the symptoms, and we consider each patient as an individual. Yes, we want to see our patient return to normal health, but "normal" for one patient may not be the same as "normal" for another. And, "normal" in the context of wholistic health may not be the same as "normal" as understood in Western medicine. For example, I believe in teaching my patients to change their way of living to avoid getting back into the same condition that caused them to seek help.

Practitioners of the drugless arts, along with their patients, will be better off if they make certain changes in the language. This will have to be a gradual process, because a language isn't made overnight. Certainly, we will keep the terms that are useful and beneficial to us. However, we will continue to add terminology that improves our ability to think and communicate clearly, and we may drop terminology that has fostered some degree of confusion or misunderstanding in the past.

THE BASIS FOR THE NEW LANGUAGE

The new language for iridology must be built around the basic foundation of iridology concepts. These are:

1.   Inherent weakness
2.   Chemical deficiencies
3.   Toxic settlements
4.   Tissue overactivity/underactivity
5.   Tissue integrity/immune system integrity

All of us have inherent weaknesses and inherent strengths as a natural part of our genetic inheritance, our native constitution. An inherent weakness appears in the iris as a section of iris fibers more widely separated from one another than the fibers in the rest of the iris. This separation of iris fibers indicates a coarser tissue structure, caused by a flawed genetic pattern in that part of the body represented by the iris.

Inherently weak tissue can be compared to coarsely or loosely woven cloth. The tissue is unable to hold the nutrients that flow into it as well as normal tissue can. Inherently weak tissue is easily depleted of nutrients and is slow in eliminating toxic metabolic wastes. This is why inherently weak organs can't keep up with normal organs in terms of activity levels or stress tolerance. They tire more easily and more often. Properly cared for, they function normally, but when inherently weak organs are over-worked or underfed, they are more easily subject to breakdown and disease than normal organs.

The breakdown of inherently weak tissue begins in either of two ways. Either depletion of needed chemical elements takes place, followed by gradual accumulation of toxic materials from the blood, lymph, and its own metabolic wastes, or else the reverse happens. If toxic wastes accumulate first because the metabolism of the organ is too slow to prevent it, tissue function is disrupted and chemical deficiencies develop. We need to understand that either chemical deficiency or toxic accumulation may come first, but the other inevitably follows, and reversal of this condition must take account of both problems.

Any abused or overworked inherent weakness end up with both chemical deficiencies and toxic accumulations. This condition, in turn, leads to an acute inflammation (overactivity), in which the irritated tissue tries to throw off the toxic material.

If suppressant drugs are used, or if the condition is neglected, the initial overactivity will run its course and underactivity will take its place. Iridology identifies four stages of inflammation: acute, subacute, chronic, and degenerative. A metabolic regression develops in that organ, gland, or tissue, which leads to successive levels of subacute, chronic, and degenerative underactivity. The toxins that contribute to this condition of underactivity also lead to congestion of the lymph system, severely impairing immune system integrity. The dominant feature of the process of progressive tissue underactivity is the loss of tissue integrity through a gradual erosion of the normal structural and functional qualities of that tissue.

For example, an iris might show chronic-to-degenerative signs in the bowel, chronic signs in the lungs and bronchials, and subacute-to-chronic signs in the pancreas, with a few nerve rings, signs of lymphatic rosary, moderate scurf rim, and underactive kidneys. We understand from this analysis that underactive elimination channels (the bowel being the most underactive and the source of most problems), are causing toxic buildups in the blood and lymph systems. This creates a general acidic condition in the body, congested lymph glands, irritated nerves, and increased stress on the pancreas.

On the basis of this information and from the patient's complaint and health history, I know what to recommend to him. I know what I need to do to take care of him, nutritionally and otherwise. There is no need to go further and talk about diseases in the tradition of Western medicine.

Some iridologists, however, might try to tell the patient that he has chronic bronchitis, a potentially cancerous condition in the bowel, and a pre-diabetic pancreas. It is my view that the iris does not reveal these things. We are not seeing disease in the iris—we are seeing levels of tissue activity that can't be translated into disease names and that can't be interpreted as particular diseases. Moreover, *we don't need to talk about diseases to be able to take care of the problem.*

The therapies or treatments used by osteopaths, chiropractors, homeopaths, acupuncturists, and other drugless practitioners are based on the interpretation of symptoms, not the diagnosis of diseases. Our therapies and treatments aim at removal of the cause of the problem, tissue correction, and restoration of tissue integrity. I realize that some of those in iridology are trying to go the way of Western medicine by "diagnosing" diseases, but I believe this is a mistake.

What are osteopaths aiming for in their diagnoses and treatments? Restoration of tissue integrity. What do chiropractors want for their patients? Restoration of tissue integrity. What do homeopaths, acupuncturists, shiatsu practitioners, herbalists, and others look for as the result of their individual therapies? Restoration of tissue integrity.

We can define tissue integrity as that state of structural cleanliness and strength that allows the highest quality of functional performance for a particular organ, gland, tissue, or individual, considering the relative positive and negative aspects of the environment. For example, a man's heart will work better and longer if his other organs are clean and functioning well than if he has an underactive liver or a toxic thyroid. Also, a person will, in general, have better health in a rural village in the mountains where the air and water are pure and the lifestyle is slower than in a city with polluted air and water. We are only as good as the tissue we are made of, and, ultimately, our tissue reflects the relative state of purity or toxicity of the environment.

THE WHOLISTIC PERSPECTIVE AND THE NEW LANGUAGE

I use the term "wholistic" rather than "holistic," because I believe we are trying to learn to treat patients in terms of "wholeness" or "the whole person"—body, mind and spirit. So, I prefer "wholistic" over "holistic."

At some level, I believe we all understand that every patient is body, mind, and spirit, and that every symptom, to some extent, touches all three aspects of our being. For example, my teacher, V.G. Rocine, believed that a person on an imbalanced diet would have mental and moral problems as well as physical problems.

The hypothalamus in the brain acts as a central relay switchboard and monitors both higher and lower nerve systems—thoughts and emotions as well as sensory, motor, sympathetic, and parasympathetic systems. The hypothalamus provides feedback to brain centers and to the endocrine system, via the pituitary gland, interacting with body systems in a two-way flow of information and participating in the healing process as well as "observing" or monitoring the activity level of every organ, gland, and tissue in the body.

In fact, I believe there is no symptom that does not reflect interaction with the body, mind, and spirit. I am not saying that a serious physical problem is either the cause or result of a serious moral problem or a serious mental problem—although it can be. We should know by now that science has linked such moral problems as unforgiveness and vengefulness with arthritis, cancer, and heart disease, just as it has linked mental problems such as worry and anxiety with ulcers and colitis.

Please understand that I am not introducing anything new when I say that every symptom involves the physical, mental, and spiritual (moral) levels. My intent is to clarify and unify our work, not to bring in any mystical or confusing ideas.

LOSS OF TISSUE INTEGRITY

The 1988 Winter Olympics in Calgary, Canada, provided a remarkable illustration of the importance of tissue integrity and the relationship between body and mind. United States speed skater Dan Jansen was favored to win in the 500-meter race the same day he received news that his sister Jane had died of complications from leukemia.

Instead of winning, however, Jansen fell on the ice as he approached the turn on the first lap of the race, his left shoe dropping only a half-inch to touch the ice before he went down. The bad news of his sister's death translated into a loss of tissue integrity that led to the fall. When a speed skater goes into a turn, there must be near-perfect coordination of arm and leg movements as the legs cross each other powerfully and crisply, the skates cutting into the ice.

Before Jansen fell, he dedicated the race to his sister. He had skated the 500-meter race before the Olympics—in practice sessions and amateur competitions—over a thousand times. His legs, like those of gold medal winner Eric Heiden in the 1980 Olympics, are massive and powerful to look at, but they didn't stand up because of the impact of the tragic news of his sister's death. Tissue integrity was compromised because of emotional pain, because of an emotional symptom.

About the fall, Jansen said, "It was so fast. I can't remember much. It felt like it slipped right out from under me and the next thing I knew, I was in the mats." Dan Jansen was also charged with a false start, something that had rarely happened before. "I was kind of confused," he said.

Amazingly, Jansen fell for a second time when he competed in the 1,000-meter race. Ahead at the time, only 200 meters from the finish line, Jansen crashed again, just as he had the previous Sunday.

Loss of Tissue Integrity Is Common

There are many other examples of loss of tissue integrity, not only among athletes but ordinary people impacted by emotional events. Fatigue takes its toll on air traffic controllers, pilots, railroad engineers, and others who bear greater-than-normal responsibilities, altering the speed of their reaction time, the acuity of their vision, and possibly their judgment, under some circumstances.

Loss of tissue integrity and related mental integrity issues may well have been involved in major U.S. train wrecks in 1987 and 1988. Tissue integrity problems are found among those who are accident prone, among drug addicts, and among men and women in prison.

In drug use, mental integrity is first compromised, then moral and physical integrity. For example, in several California communities, women have been jailed for trading sex for cocaine. They have been responsible for a sharp increase in sexually-transmitted diseases.

The tragic death of Elvis Presley, I believe, was due to his trying to live up to the expectations of others and stay on top in his singing career with the help of drugs. The sad fact is that drugs always lead to physical, mental, and moral loss of integrity.

What Do We Mean by "Integrity"?

Perhaps we will gain a better understanding of the reason I am proposing a new language for iridology and other alternative health arts if I include the analogy of what we consider "integrity" in a person. When you have known a person for a while, how do you describe that person's level of integrity?

Integrity of the behavior can never really be separated from the integrity of mind and morals. Integrity tends to flow from wholeness, completeness, the proper integration and working of each part with all the others. In one sense, a man can only be as good as his bowel activity, but even if a man's bowel is working well, that doesn't necessarily mean his whole body is functioning with integrity (although chances are high that it is). In turn, the bowel condition, and many other parts of the body, depends on the food regimen and lifestyle of a person.

The importance of each organ, gland, and tissue of the whole body emphasizes the need to treat the whole body, no matter what disease, ailment, or malfunction is present. That is why we can't just treat symptoms. Similarly, we must take into account thoughts, attitudes, emotions, behaviors, and beliefs that may be affecting the patient's condition. What goes on in the mind affects the body; what goes on in the body affects the mind. Both contribute to any disease, ailment, or malfunction.

Challenges to Integrity

Today there are great challenges to the whole concept of integrity. Most of these challenges are the result of chemical and drug pollution throughout the world.

Everywhere we look, we find chemicals. Acid rain in parts of the United States and Canada, caused by industrial pollution of the air, is poisoning streams, rivers, and lakes, killing fish and other wildlife. Auto pollution in urban areas is pumping carcinogens into peoples' lungs.

Our drinking water is also polluted. Even the Environmental Protection Agency admits that industrial chemicals can enter and contaminate our drinking water. Among the chemicals that can be found in our drinking water are asbestos, chlorine, flourine, colloidal matter, detergents, hydrocarbons, pesticides, pyrogens, radioactive chemicals, and elements such as sodium, calcium, magnesium, cadmium, and others.

Chemical additives and toxic spray residues are in our food. Sulfide sprays are on many of the foods at salad bars. We put chemicals on our skin to smell good or to help us get a suntan or to block out the sun's rays. Who knows what adverse chemical reactions take place when the ultraviolet in sunlight interacts with chemicals on our skin? Agent Orange, a chemical defoliant used during the Vietnam War, has been a disabling blight in the lives of all who came in contact with it, both United States servicemen and the Vietnamese people.

Television ads brainwash people about the "virtues" of drugs, and each year, millions of people pollute their bodies with tons of prescription and nonprescription drugs. In prisons, 90 percent of the inmates have used drugs—marijuana, cocaine, heroin, uppers, downers—you name it. Our hospitals and nursing homes and convalescent homes have become drug-dispensing centers.

We must realize that using drugs—any drugs—or getting too many chemical substances in our bodies results in loss of tissue integrity, mental integrity, and eventually, moral integrity.

I want to briefly clarify what I mean by moral integrity. Moral integrity requires, I believe, that we consider the impact of our own decisions and behaviors on the lives of others. It also requires that we be willing to change if we see we are harming anyone. In a nutshell, moral integrity means living by the golden rule: "Do unto others as you would have them do unto you." I believe we are all born to serve and uplift one another, not to bring harm to others.

THE WAYS OF WESTERN MEDICINE

If we consider the ideas of Western medicine about disease and cure as compared with the perspective of alternative health arts such as homeopathy, chiropractic, osteopathy, naturopathy, herbology, acupuncture, nutrition, and iridology, we find some distinct differences that must be reflected in the new language.

With some exception, few drugless practitioners claim to treat disease. Most treat tissue conditions as revealed through symptoms and reflex conditions. They look for reversal of symptoms, cleansing of tissue, remineralization, and restoration and correction of tissue. They try to teach patients not to abuse areas of inherent weakness in the body that led to the problem in the first place.

In contrast, Western medicine, guided by its classification of disease and a broad array of tests, treats the maladies it discovers with vaccines, drugs, radiation, and surgery. There is no reversal of disease. Instead, there is an apparent attempt to blot out the disease with drugs or therapies as dangerous as the disease itself. Drugs have undesirable side effects, long-term effects, and time-bomb effects. A whole new branch of Western medicine is called iatrogenic medicine, and its job is to correct serious health problems caused by drugs or other treatments. Iatrogenic diseases are caused by the treatments given by Western medicine.

THE PRIORITIES OF IRIDOLOGY

There is a major issue here—the issue of priorities. Common sense, respect for the individual, and concern for health care quality would seem to dictate that our treatment of choice would always start with the least dangerous, least traumatic treatment appropriate for the patient and his condition. You wouldn't prescribe herbal tea for someone who had just suffered a major coronary, but it might be best for a person with a mild digestive upset. There are people with chronic diseases for whom I believe we should consider the reversal process, cleansing of toxins, and the healing crisis. The reversal process involves remineralization and other treatments until a healing crisis occurs, which provides the cleansing of toxic deposits and the restoration of tissue integrity. Many of us in the drugless art believe this is what treatment is all about. Our language must reflect such distinctions.

To determine tissue integrity, we can ask these questions: Is the tissue performing its function correctly? Are the tissues impaired that normally depend on that particular tissue? Is there an absence of abnormal symptoms? Does it appear normal in the iris? Does the patient report any symptoms that lead us to expect the iris to show problems? Are the person's diet and lifestyle conducive to wellness? Does the person show integrity in the way he or she lives? We should expect that integrity in the larger context will include integrity in its "parts," so to speak.

The connection between the moral, mental, and physical aspects of the body can be shown this way: if a man thinks cheerful thoughts (mental), he will act cheerful and friendly toward people (moral). This good thinking will, in turn, result in responsible, balanced tissues and organs (physical).

A man who thinks greedy thoughts will practice "greedy" behavior, and his body will suffer physically. Because he is greedy he may overeat, have excessive sexual desire, and hurt others to get what he wants.

Is mental integrity derived from physical tissue integrity? That's like asking, "Which came first, the chicken or the egg?" The mind and body are interactive—each influences the other. How we think and speak are extremely important. A neurosurgeon has pointed out that if Broca's speech center is affected or weakened, the weakness not only affects other senses but weakens our will power, our assertiveness, our ability to "be in charge." That's why most us need to let go of critical, negative speaking and learn to speak health, wholeness, success, and prosperity. We need to speak the best about others and forget their bad points. Obviously, how we think and talk influences our emotions; we can talk ourselves up or down. This is another reason why it is so important for the natural healing arts to have their own language.

How we talk about what we do—or do not do—determines our mindset toward our patients, ourselves, and our health care objectives. Keep in mind what I mentioned in the previous paragraph about Broca's speech center. If you want to work toward tissue integrity, you will have to think and speak the language of tissue integrity. Language affects goals. Language influences the means we choose to achieve our health care objectives.

What about the issue of ethics? Does the issue of ethics involve integrity? Of course it does! To some extent, language can be thought of as a food. We are affected by what we say, as we are affected by what we eat. Thought—and speech—forms channels for energy. Energy gives power to ideas, which help structure the way we live.

In a way, I feel that the life-energy moves from the spirit to the soul (or mind) and from the mind to the body, carrying the moral directives into the mental, the mental directives into the body. The body, so motivated and inspired, then naturally moves to carry out the directives and instructions given to it. Isn't this wonderful? On the other hand, the physical energy supplied by our food regimen and sleep habits first energizes the body, then flows to the brain, and finally flows from the mind to the spirit.

The physical, mental, and moral dimensions energize and influence one another constantly and have a tremendous effect on our health. Usually, all three are moving toward health or all three are moving away from health. They are integrated with one another and they are all dynamic, moving, constantly influencing and driving toward goals of one sort or another.

When the body, mind, and morals are balanced and in tune with one another, we have perseverance, stamina, and energy for the long haul to success. On the other hand, if we turn in the other direction, we find that the same pathway that leads "downhill" through the symptoms and tissue activity stages of acute, subacute, chronic, and degenerative levels also includes a mental and moral downhill tendency. We need to acknowledge this in our language.

Anything that affects one organ in the body affects them all, while anything that affects the body also affects the mind and spirit. A living organism is an integrated, interdependent, inseparable set of related parts, and a lowering of function in any part cuts into the others. There is, in this sense, a unity of function.

No one is justified in being criminal. The lack of moral integrity indicates integrity losses at the mental and physical levels as well, but the universal human need is to be justified, to be aligned with integrity. Integrity is the "norm," so to speak, and there is a deep hunger inside of each person to express integrity.

In May of 1987, *Time* magazine's cover featured the question "What Ever Happened to ETHICS?" The cover story discussed how hypocrisy, betrayal, and greed are dragging America down as Wall Street brokers and investors, television evangelists, politicians, high-ranking government officials, and many other Americans in unprecedented numbers have been caught in criminal acts or morally-compromising situations.

Integrity is very much a choice—a choice to be normal, yes, but also a choice to be the best possible individual that we were created to be. Health is more than a physical condition, and we need a language that constantly affirms the priority and importance of integrity at all levels of life.

We need a new language to describe the basic assumptions of the natural healing art. No doubt we will keep the concepts of acute, subacute, chronic, and degenerative, but we need to remove our focus from the idea of disease. We need to think in terms of symptoms, in terms of level of activity, in terms of potential and actual loss of tissue integrity.

Our new language must include Hering's law, which says, "All cure comes from the head down, from the inside out and in reverse order as symptoms have appeared." In my books *Iridology I* and *Iridology II*, I have described the reversal process by which Hering's law leads to the healing crisis, and many in the healing arts are familiar with this teaching.

We want to describe the healing crisis with a language that talks about building toward tissue integrity.

The Good Book talks about becoming a "new person." This should be the goal we teach our patients to work toward—a new person, a person of integrity, with that integrity evident at the physical, mental, and moral levels of life.

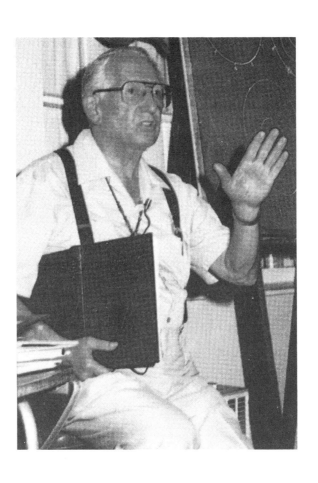

CHAPTER 3
Advanced Iridology

Many practitioners in the health arts who use iridology have asked me, "What do you see in the future for iridology? What advances are on the horizon?" Other health professionals—more recently introduced to iridology as a diagnostic aid—ask, "What's the bottom line in iridology? Can it make an important difference in my practice?" I want to try to answer these questions in this chapter, because I'm really excited about the future of iridology.

A DIAGNOSTIC OVERVIEW

I don't know of a single test or battery of tests that can show what's going on inside the body as well as iridology does. In the future, I think computerized iridology is going to be widely used to help correlate and interpret all the other tests doctors use—x-rays, blood tests, urinalyses, electroencephalography, electrocardiograms, and even sonograms, Nuclear Magnetic Resonance imaging, and infrared analyses.

What's the first thing an explorer does when trying to find his way around uncharted territory? He looks for a high place, a promontory, and climbs up to get an overview of where things are. He sees the river, swamps, hills, canyons, trees, and other features of the landscape, and where they are in relation to one another. Then he is able to climb down and investigate individual characteristics of the area and fit them into the "big picture."

Medical tests are like individual parts of a landscape. Let's say the blood test is "the river," the urinalysis is the "swamp," and the x-ray shows "canyons and trees." The doctor still doesn't know where all these things are in relation to one another.

Iridology can help tie these tests together and make sense of patient symptoms, showing which parts of the body are most in need of care and what the source of the problem is in many cases. This will be a tremendous help in establishing priorities for any treatment program.

THE OFFICE VISIT

Before we discuss the future of iridology, let's get a clear picture of what the iridologist is doing now.

No patient ever comes into the doctor's office with only one problem. As mentioned before, one toxic organ can affect the whole body. The toxic organ can trigger secondary reflex conditions in many parts of the body, and often the patient's complaints are concerned with these secondary problems, not the basic cause.

I use iridology to find out which parts of the patient's body appear to be most chronic. This is done by comparing the degree of darkness in iris lesions throughout the eye. The darkest lesions always indicate the oldest, most chronic, or degenerative inflammations. This tells us what is most likely the source of other troubles.

After the iris analysis, I ask for the main complaint and fill out a patient history, which includes operations and other prior health problems. Often, what is going on in a person's body may date back to some condition that was not properly taken care of twenty years ago, perhaps even back in childhood.

Once the patient's history is covered, I consider the most chronic conditions to be the highest priority. Tissue cannot rejuvenate or rebuild in a toxic body, so the first thing that must be done is to clean up the body and bloodstream. A polluted body cannot repair itself. We can founder in our own toxins as underactive bowels absorb toxic materials through the bowel wall, contaminating the blood, which carries this unwanted material to the inherently weak tissues. This will cause low-grade infections to develop, sapping vitality.

During the first visit, it is important to start the patient on a correction program, a new path. The patient's body is in its present condition because the body has molded to the old lifestyle, with its undesirable habits. We have to go back and straighten this out, because this lifestyle has produced a warped body, and certain organs are starved of the chemical elements they need.

It is necessary to realize that you can't take the right chemical elements from even the purest, most wholesome foods and expect to take care of toxic-laden tissue. Toxic-laden tissue is too underactive to put nutrients to good use. So, we concentrate on cleansing first.

The first step in cleansing is to consider the elimination channels, because toxins could not build up in the body if they were being properly eliminated. The organs of elimination are the bowel, kidneys, lymphatic system, lungs, and skin, and in the majority of patients I have examined, the eyes show the bowel and bronchial areas of the body to be in the darkest, most chronic condition. When the organs of elimination are toxic-laden, the body is in trouble. It doesn't matter whether the source of the toxins is improper diet or failure of the body to rid itself of metabolic wastes; in either case, we have to stop breaking down before we can start building up.

Toxic material in the bowel is often responsible for neck aches, running ears, allergies, and poor circulation. Kidney disturbances can be helped by taking care of the bowel. The same is true of the lungs and bronchials, which we associate with so many catarrhal conditions—bronchitis, hay fever, asthma, colds, and flus. If the skin is a problem, there are things we can do to help. For each elimination channel, there are both nutritional and mechanical methods of treatment.

Patients need to be taught that diseases are not "caught" and not "cured." Our bodies mold to what we do. We eat, drink, work, and play disease into existence. If a person is not interested in living differently—I'd like to say *correctly*—to bring his body back to a state of well-being through healthful living, then there is nothing I can do for him. Every patient must choose between Nature's way and the way of nostrums and suppressive drugs.

My first visit with a patient requires a great deal of sincerity and cooperation. With those elements, healing can begin to take place.

There may be other things we can do during the first visit. For example, herb teas will help take care of some immediate aches and pains, some local problems. However, if the symptoms are caused by the long-term development of a condition, there is no alternative but to go back and straighten it out. I do this by putting these patients on a cleansing program and what I call my "Health and Harmony Food Regimen" and any supplements they may particularly need.

Many people need a good talking to; many people need to change their attitudes. The marriage or job may be contributing to the problem, as may a long-suppressed desire to develop or express some talent or gift. But you can only cover so much during that first visit, and it is best to stick to nutrition at first. After all, no one can be expected to think sweet thoughts on a sour stomach. A good "house cleaning" is the correct way to begin.

THE HIGHEST PRIORITY: UNDERSTANDING THE BRAIN

The most important organ in the body is the brain, but the brain is the least understood organ in iridology. If we look at the iridology map of the iris (Figure 3.1), we see that the upper portion from 11 o'clock to 1 o'clock in both irides is devoted to the brain. The brain is like a symphony conductor, directing and overseeing all of the parts of the body, coordinating each part or instrument with all the others to produce the harmonious and exciting performance we call "life."

Most of the iridology chart is mapped out in terms of anatomy. Each labelled area corresponds to that part of the body. The area that corresponds to the brain, however, is not mapped out in terms of anatomy, except for the pituitary gland, pineal gland, and the medulla. Instead, the brain area is subdivided into symmetrical slices that are named mostly after brain and mental faculties and functions, with a couple of psychotic states (obsession and hallucination) added for good measure. I think we can all agree that the area of the brain on the iridology chart needs further investigation and development.

The brain is of great importance to iridology because it plays a major role in maintaining the health of the whole body. For that reason, proper brain care must be one of our highest health priorities. Anything that happens to reduce the efficiency of the brain (or any of its parts) not only alters our perception of reality and flow of consciousness, but usually impairs one or more body functions. For example, impotence and loss of interest in sex is a frequent consequence of drug and alcohol abuse.

I believe we are only beginning to understand how delicate and important brain/mind activities are. It is my opinion that what is going on in the minds of the mother and father at the time of conception will affect the future of their child. This is another reason why advanced iridology must emphasize brain care.

We need to be able to increase the amount of useful health-related information we can get from the brain area of the iris. This will come in the future, I am sure, from the work of some of the bright young iridologists around the world.

Recognizing Risks to Brain/Mind Health

If the brain is not fed properly, it cannot function properly. The morality of the generation to come will be determined in part by how we take care of our brains and mental faculties today. Our culture is allowing destructive processes to take place that will reduce the brain/mind inheritance of the next generation. I use the term "brain/mind" to acknowledge that there is such constant interaction between the physical and the mental in the context of discussing health that it makes better sense to combine them.

One way our culture contributes to the breakdown of the brain/mind faculty is through drug use. The mental faculties of women are said to be reduced by as much as 10 percent from the use of oral contraceptives. The federal government says that if pregnant mothers drink alcoholic beverages, brain damage may occur in their unborn babies. The same risk applies to pregnant women who are drug addicts.

Few people understand that drugs and alcohol can cause genetic damage in either parent long before conception. This genetic damage can be passed on to the unborn child years later. Drugs and alcohol should be avoided, period.

Drugs have undesirable side effects, long-term effects, and time-bomb effects. Do people keep track of how much aspirin or phenacetin they've taken? No. Every drug affects the brain and body in abnormal, unnatural ways, yet we don't limit ourselves or keep track of what we're doing. The drugs each generation takes may very well affect several subsequent generations through genetic damage affecting the brain and psoric taints—genetically transmitted tissue damage in the body. Iridology, more than any other form of analysis, will help us trace these things.

There are many unfortunate habits that people today indulge in. They include the use of junk foods, candy, chewing gum, soft drinks, and cigarettes. There are poisons among the thousands of chemical food additives so commonly used today. If a substance is not toxic of itself, it may become toxic when it combines with old drug residues in the tissues or with other chemical substances in the bowel.

Drugs tend to settle more in one brain area than in another. Their effects on endocrine glands cause hormonal abnormalities and cause damage to genetic patterns to such an extent that we can hardly expect to have normal children. We all want the perfect child, but our chances of having one are getting smaller.

My teacher, V.G. Rocine, told me that at one time a young lady came to him and asked, "What do I need to do to have a healthy baby?" She was five months pregnant and wanted to make sure that she had a healthy child, mentally and physically. Rocine told her, "My dear, you should have come to me twenty years ago!" Perfection is not an overnight task but a life-long program. When we persist in habits and behaviors that diminish our own health level, we steal from the health of the next generation, because virtually everything we do can influence the genetic and mental inheritance of our children.

We must do the best we can with the mental faculties that we have. Iridology can help us with this. If we could build up, by proper feeding, the cerebellum, the midbrain, the cerebrum, the nervous system, and the glandular system of children from the time of their birth, we wouldn't have so many inherent weaknesses. We could have a new generation.

Iridology is the only science we have that will show the inherent weaknesses in a body. The locations of the weaknesses are well written in the iris. If we take care of our inherent weaknesses today, we won't have to pass them along to the next generation. These inherent weaknesses will produce weaknesses in the next generation if we ignore them, or if we take up destructive habits or neglect proper food habits.

We have to overfeed our inherently weak organs, glands, and tissues and keep them very clean. Unless we overfeed the inherent weaknesses, they tend not to get enough of the chemical elements they need. If we are careful, our inherently weak tissues remain healthy and active. Then, the

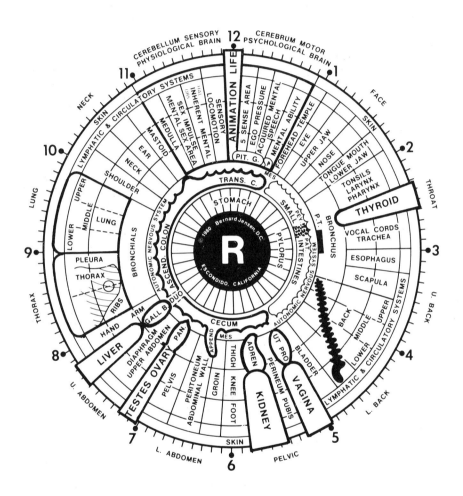

RIGHT IRIS
P — Pineal
Pey Pat — Peyers Patches
Mes — Mesentery
Hal — Hallucination
P.T. — Parathyroid

Figure 3.1   Chart to Iridology

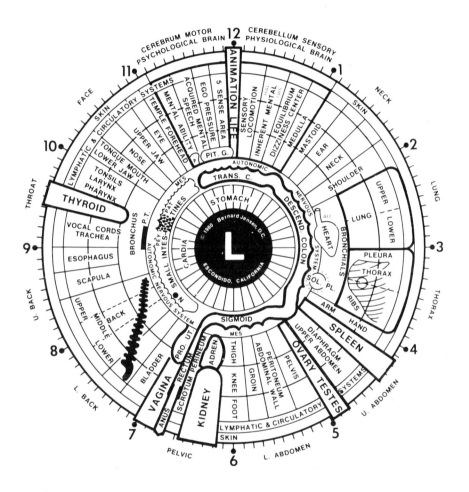

LEFT IRIS
Pit. G. — Pituitary Gland
Sol. Pl. — Solar Plexus
N — Navel
Obs — Obsession
AO — Aorta

next generation will not inherit these weaknesses. This is advanced iridology.

Even Nobel Prize winners, who may be geniuses in one field, have some kind of inherent weakness in the body. Advanced iridology will try to help people become totally healthy, in mind, body, and spirit, because it is not only mental genius we need. It is people who are strong and healthy in all aspects of mind and body. We need to encourage people to avoid the destructive aspects of life that are breaking down their bodies as well as society.

We want people who are capable of winning the Nobel Prize and who are moral people as well. We want people who are not interested in carrying on weaknesses like cravings and out-of-control behaviors that break down our society rather than build it up.

THE ADVANTAGES OF IRIDOLOGY

Many people have expressed the desire to study advanced applications of iridology. I learned the advantages of using iridology the hard way, by first trying to use nutrition to heal people without any way of identifying inherently weak tissues or knowing exactly what foods to give them.

I learned to use nutrition systematically for healing from V.G. Rocine, before I began to practice iridology. Dr. Rocine used a complex theory of chemical types of people to analyze nutritional needs. Then he would custom-design a diet for each patient. My book *The Chemistry of Man* further explains Rocine's methods.

Many times I've had to use Rocine's chemical types to find out what foods would correct the conditions of people who came to me for help. Rocine was able to determine what foods are necessary to treat a particular deficiency. Hippocrates, too, was able to treat his patients with foods. Rocine found that in feeding his patients the right foods, he could change some of the adverse health conditions that developed in the body.

Once I began to understand iridology, a whole new world opened up to me. I could see which parts of the body were inherently weak, and I knew what chemical elements were needed by each part. I also knew what chemical elements were in each food. Designing a diet for correction of some health problem became as easy as adding two and two to get four.

Iridology is an analysis that tells us how we can bring our bodies back to normal. Iridology reveals the way we have built our bodies, the way we have developed tissue underactivities, mineral deficiencies, and toxic settlements in the tissues. From this information, it is an easy step to figure out the chemical elements necessary to take care of deficiencies. Iridology reveals the parts of the body that will break down under abuse long before any problems or symptoms actually develop. Knowing this, we can see how to keep a body healthy by taking the right preventive measures before breakdown occurs. All you need is iridology and a cooperative spirit.

We need a means of keeping us on the path, some way of showing that our health program is working. We need to show that inflammations may flare up in the acute stage, but through proper care we can restore the body to balance and health.

The subacute, chronic, and degenerative stages of disease develop when a person suppresses symptoms through treatment and use of over-the-counter and prescription drugs. Iridology can show these taking place.

The American Cancer Society tells us that it takes twenty years or more to build some kinds of cancer! It takes twenty years to build a certain kind of person! When a person has inherent weaknesses and doesn't live properly, he is going to end up with certain diseases and glandular imbalances that may lead to genetic breakdowns in sperm or ova. Iridology can identify these symptoms before they reach the acute stage, and treat them with the right foods.

IRIDOLOGY CAN HELP BRING A BETTER GENERATION

With genetic weaknesses passed along to the next generation, we are going to develop abnormal children, problem children, and handicapped children. Advanced iridology can be a tool to help us work toward cleanliness in the body. The iridologist can see effects of thalidomide. He will help mothers-to-be in their pregnancies so that their children don't lack arms and legs when they are born. Presently, we are taking care of deformed children after they are born.

Why shouldn't we take care of that problem before it happens? Why shouldn't we start taking care of these things? We can do this by seeing what is in the iris.

The advanced iridologist should help make sure that the new generation is not going to carry on the weaknesses that have built up in their forefathers. Our forefathers had their problems. They had to take care of many diseases.

Diseases, ailments, and sicknesses haven't just started in recent years. Some conditions, like arthritis, began thousands of years ago. But drug problems are more recent. Iridology shows the effects of drugs. Everyone is looking for a drug that will bring a cure. Yet, you can search through a thousand prescriptions and not find a single drug that is capable of correcting abnormal tissue. The true correction will be brought out through nutrition.

The advanced iridologist must adhere to procedures that promote tissue purity, procedures that work for cleanliness, wholeness, and restoration. We cannot expect the next generation to be well or expect the inherent weaknesses to leave our bodies unless we take the right steps for correction now.

Iridology could be a great help in finding what inherent weaknesses will be passed down from the parents to the children. When we take this knowledge, express it, put it in writing, and share it, we can take steps to help people raise healthy children.

DEVELOPING BALANCE IN THE BODY

In studying with Dr. Rocine over a period of years, I was interested in his discovery of the different "chemical" types of people. He believed that people developed into recognizably different chemical types (i.e., "sodium type," "calcium type," etc.) over the years through a chronic lack of certain chemical elements and an overabundance of other chemical elements in their diets.

Some people have great difficulty digesting or assimilating foods so that they can get the minerals they need to improve themselves physically. There are people who have difficulty in repairing and rebuilding. Some seem to retain drug settlements they have accumulated over the years.

Through proper chemical feeding, however, we can take care of the inherent weaknesses in the body so they cannot be passed from one generation to another. We can clean up the tissues by a balanced feeding program developed through the use of iridology.

Some people have tissues that readily absorb and hold drugs. Other people do not have this problem. They seem to be carrying what I call "drug imprints" from past generations. Their immunity to certain diseases has been lost as these drug imprints have been carried from one generation to another. Somewhere in their family tree, predecessors used heavy doses of drugs to suppress one or more diseases. The drugs affect their genetic structure and produce a type of tissue that behaves as though it carries drug residues. Such tissue is sensitive, irritable, and vulnerable to disease. Homeopaths call such conditions "miasms." Rocine categorized such people as "medeic types" and developed a program for cleansing and rebuilding the drug-encumbered tissue. Iridology shows the miasmic eye to be murky, dark, clouded—like muddy water.

Iridology is meant for the advanced thinker, for the person who would like to take care of health problems that drugs can't solve, problems that Western medicine doesn't have the answer to.

In iridology, we can see how to balance the activity of one organ with another. It is an entirely different system of analyzing than Western medicine utilizes. Western medicine has concentrated on cataloging diseases and their symptoms and, correspondingly, cataloging drugs and treatments for specific diseases or specific aspects of a disease. In treating diabetes with insulin, for example, we neglect to take care of the twenty or so other things wrong that usually accompany diabetes.

This practice has to be changed in the future. There is no one whose inherent weaknesses have led to diabetes who doesn't also need to take care of the bowel. We should try to break up inherent weaknesses so they aren't carried on to the next generation—for example, passing along a predisposition for diabetes to our children.

Most doctors agree that those born with inherent weaknesses are difficult to cure. They are the ones who have the most difficulty getting well. Diabetics who acquire their problem at the age of forty or fifty are often able to overcome it because they were born with a fairly good pancreas.

It would be wise if we realized, in treating various conditions in the body, that everyone has inherent weaknesses. It is in these inherent weaknesses that toxic settlements develop. After mineral deficiencies have weakened a particular organ, gland, or tissue, toxic material begins to accumulate because there is no power to throw it off. This gland or organ may become unproductive. A gland may be poor, possibly too imbalanced for reproduction and too weak to allow us to perform our jobs properly. A weak gland may sensitize us to the extent that we develop an antipathy to the climate. Allergies develop that may preclude us from living in certain parts of the country. We may have to move to the mountains or to the desert. The problem, of course, goes back to inherent weaknesses brought down through generations. We have to take care of them, or there is no improvement in health. Iridology is the advanced science that can help us do this.

The main thing to consider in an iridology reading is that we generally do not find one chronic condition developing. There are ordinarily five to eight chronic conditions simultaneously developing in various parts of the body. No one comes into this world without several inherent weaknesses, and these weak organs cannot get rid of toxic settlements. So, when we find one chronic organ, we always look for more, as the toxic settlements take over one organ after another.

When we find one degenerative stage in an organ, there are usually other organs that have developed degenerative conditions as well. People seldom die from one disease. There is no condition that cannot be found in the iris that doesn't have as many as fifteen related conditions, fifteen other parts of the body that also have inherent weaknesses, toxic settlements, and mineral deficiencies. Every underactive organ tends to drag down the rest of the body.

Even in cases of AIDS, people don't die from AIDS proper. They die from the AIDS-related diseases. They die from pneumonia or hemorrhages of the bowel. They die from bronchial troubles and lung disorders—respiratory breakdown. They die from kidney disorders or Bright's disease (nephritis).

When the skin, an eliminative organ, is not working properly, it will be a drag on every other organ in the body. Dry, inactive skin that is not perspiring and getting rid of toxic material is associated with other inherent weaknesses in the body. This can prevent the body from being clean, pure, and whole. We cannot properly alleviate skin problems unless we take care of the skin as an eliminative organ.

A recent news article quoted university researchers as recognizing that the skin is an eliminative organ of significant value, as important as the bowel, kidneys, lungs, and bronchials. Near-surface blood vessels and lymph vessels release liquid metabolic wastes that penetrate the pores of the skin as perspiration and evaporate into the air. As much waste is eliminated through the skin in a day's time as is eliminated through the bowel.

To take care of a person properly we must understand that organ problems may be related to one another. Health professionals see the symptoms coming from one organ when the cause actually is in another organ. For example, if stomach cancer is found, it is cut out. Then lung cancer is found so it is cut out, too. Finally, after two operations, the cause of the stomach and the lung cancers is found—cancer of the colon. This is where it all started and where the first treatment should have been. We must catch on to these things and learn more about prevention and early detection and treatment.

NUTRITION CAN REPLACE OLD TISSUE WITH NEW TISSUE

The only cure Western medicine has for cancer, in most cases, is cutting it out. What they do not realize is that anyone with cancer also has many other conditions that should be taken care of. But, unfortunately, they do not find these other problems so the person can be treated more wholistically. Such a person will never be cured until integrity is restored to the rest of the inherently weak tissues that have toxic settlements and mineral deficiencies.

A person may think he is in good health. He may tell everyone that he feels good, but is actually one of those that the medical profession talks about when it reports that two out of ten people who say they are "feeling good" have at least one chronic disease developing in their body.

Iridology advocates a health philosophy of cleanliness, emphasizing approaches to health that will purify the polluted bodies of people who live in industrialized cultures. Why should we ignore the relationship between health and cleanliness? The importance of cleanliness has been stated by Hippocrates, Rocine, Otto Carque, John Tilden, and many others who healed people with foods and herbs.

It is time that all those in all the healing arts who are interested in the purity and good of the human body get together. This is what we should work for.

Advanced iridology is going to help the acupuncturist. Advanced iridology is going to help the chiropractor. Iridology is going to help the osteopath. The iridologist is trying to put the type of diagnosis together that Rocine hoped to develop. Advanced iridology will help everyone in the healing arts.

A FUTURE LOOK AT IRIDOLOGY

Where is advanced iridology going? We must take the basic concepts of iridology and apply them together with the right therapies to make sure that we are getting rid of inflammations in the body. We should go through the entire body, taking care of all suppressed conditions, whether they are from junk food, pills, ill-thinking, or depleted and enervated nerves. Those who know enough about iridology will be able to improvise useful applications to health care problems no matter what their areas of specialization are in the health arts.

Hippocrates would be happy to see that we can now show that there are certain foods that are good for certain conditions in the body. Iridologists are not just saying "a prune is a good laxative." We are saying that foods have individual properties that provide the individual chemical elements needed by each organ, gland and tissue.

Any day now, the computer is going to be able to coordinate iris analysis with a proper remedial diet. It is almost an impossibility for many to remember all the foods containing these chemical elements, the qualities they have, and the way they should be applied to correct health problems. But, a computer can be used as an "extra brain" that can keep all this in its memory. The smart man of the future will use the computer as a consultant that will help him devise exactly the right healing program.

EVALUATING FUTURE HEALTH PROSPECTS

In the future, the Army and Navy can use iridology to evaluate who would be the best kind of person to have a career in the military. Who is capable? What kind of constitution do they have? Are they going to have the necessary stamina? Is this person going to have the energy and the power to carry on? Is he or she going to have to drop out in a few years?

This will be the job of the advanced iridologist. The day is coming when the iridologist will be able to prove that the cell structure in the iris of the eye accurately signals tissue conditions elsewhere in the human body and its organs. We will find that in certain jobs, a certain type of person is going to fail because of inherent weaknesses. The advanced iridologist is going to be able to warn a person in time to prevent that inherent weakness from breaking down.

The advanced iridologist will have a place in the development of managers and business executives—people whose training normally takes many years.

A hotel owner was telling me about three men who, through years of training, had become valuable employees because of hotel management skills. But, one died; the second was scheduled for an operation; and the third became so sick he could no longer stay on the job. These men spent years training to become managers, and then ended up with serious health problems. The employer who wants his employees to be as healthy as possible will look to the iridologist for this kind of information.

I had the privilege of talking to a man who owns a large computer company. He said that his secretary had eye trouble and was told that she would not be able to see again out of one of her eyes. The owner applied some of the teachings that he had learned from my work, and suggested to his secretary that she eat certain mineral-rich foods. She did, and her eyesight returned.

The employer of the future is going to use the iridologist to keep his employees well and keep them on the job. He should install a "food bar" so that his employees can get the best possible foods. Carrot juices, special teas, and special health-building snacks should be available.

Employees should not be exposed to rest break risks such as the "pause that refreshes" (referring to cola drinks). Soft drinks, sweets, coffee, and donuts will eventually cause health breakdowns. Many companies and employers are paying temporary employees. They are not employing people who feel it is a privilege to work because they are in good health, who want to work because they are in good health, and will be there a long time because they are in good health.

The advanced iridologist has a big job to do in the future. Right now it is an "undiscovered" science, but it will be discovered in the future, so that all of these conditions can change.

Is man's consciousness ready to accept this? Many times people balk at accepting a new thing that will change their way of living. They are not ready for purity. They are not ready for higher consciousness. They are not ready to accept those things that can lead to a better life.

Do people who are getting married really want to have healthy children? Would they undergo counseling and treatment for a year to have them? What does a parent think will happen if their child is born seriously deficient in health and ability? Do they think the child will have a good life and be productive? Yes, any handicapped person can learn to accept greater limits than others, but it is a shame when the handicap was unnecessary in the first place.

Changes in consciousness will make changes in the physical body. Willpower and comprehension will enable us to focus our thoughts and follow a more single path. We have to be willing to work toward a clean body, one that does not have toxic settlements or mineral deficiencies. When is a person going to take on this consciousness?

This consciousness is found when a person is dedicated to iridology, for he is the one who is out there teaching that type of program. He believes in it. He is trying to uplift other people. He recognizes that people are born to grow and serve and uplift others. He adopts a new philosophy that is born out of the possibilities that are revealed in iridology.

Those who are devoting themselves to iridology and practicing it with a good heart and higher consciousness are those who are going to bring something wonderful to the human race, something to live for in the future. It won't be a doomsday program. People are beginning to look for an alternative, and part of the answer can be iridology. We need iridologists who will uplift and change the human race and help us work toward healthy bodies.

The advanced iridologist will take a different view of incidents such as the Bhopal tragedy in India a few years ago. Thousands of people were overcome or killed due to a toxic gas leak in a nearby Union Carbide plant. It is a crime that people have to suffer because of the manufacture of poisonous sprays and artificial fertilizers and drugs that are doing more harm than good in the first place. This is degrading to the human race, and we can do something about it.

One summer in California 10,000,000 watermelons contaminated with a toxic chemical had to be destroyed. In the Far East a few years back, thousands died from eating seed grain coated with a toxic chemical to protect it from insects and rodents.

I'm not sure this generation will fully understand the damage caused by the chemical, Agent Orange, that was used in Vietnam. The deadly effects of this chemical may go on for several generations. Iridology tells us that these things should be prevented altogether.

Why doesn't man recognize that he is making our oceans and lakes unfit for fish to swim in and live in? Foods today have become carriers of drugs, bringing on taints that our next generation is going to have to take care of. We are developing a miasmic population—people so drug-ridden that their tissues are difficult to repair and rebuild. They are people who tend to attract disease and illness.

CAN IRIDOLOGY CHANGE TOMORROW'S NEWS?

At speeds up to fifty miles an hour, a runaway train and six locomotives barreled through a thirty mile stretch of Massachusetts. The train stopped when dispatchers were able to switch the train onto sidings, where it crashed into empty boxcars. The runaway train was blamed on labor troubles. Investigators said the train was set in motion deliberately.

Is it possible that we have people who can be so malicious? Such people are sick and in need of treatment. They have gone too long with an ill body and mental problems. They are ailing and need treatment, and it is possible that we don't recognize it.

Iridology can recognize the signs of mental stress and mental breakdown. We are going to have to take care of these people.

Not long ago in Media, Pennsylvania, a lady admitted that she murdered her two-and-a-half year old son because he was born with brain damage. Why should she have a brain damaged child? What was the cause of this? The advanced iridologist should be there to help take care of that.

The mother's action was blamed on stress. Her child had to go through therapy, and this eventually wore the mother out. I can imagine what it must have been like caring for that child day after day. The child's leg motion was severely restricted. He had to be tended to every twenty minutes for twelve hours every day. This is too much for any mother.

What would the advanced iridologist do with this case? If he could study cases like this, see what the eye shows, and write it up, he might be able to help.

Doctors report that six months after Barney Clark had his heart transplant he contracted pneumonia. Where were his inherent weaknesses? Can these doctors tell? Were they able to see the lack of integrity of the lung tissue? Could they see that he was headed for pneumonia? As he got over pneumonia, he developed nephritis—kidney trouble. How long did his kidney trouble exist before it manifested itself? Barney Clark died some months later of bowel toxemia.

The doctors' reports state that a person should never have a heart transplant unless he is healthy. Who decides whether we are healthy or not? Only the advanced iridologist can show that ill health begins in a child. It is through symptom suppression that chronic diseases are acquired.

THE IRIDOLOGIST AS TEACHER

The iridologist has a big job to do. That is, to go out and teach that the prevention of disease is the most important thing that we have to take care of in the process of human development. This prevention of disease should start in our homes and schools.

Why don't schools teach avoidance of alcohol? They show the effects of drugs and how they produce addicts, and even show how they treat addiction. But children should be educated and motivated to say no to drugs.

We have to develop a right consciousness in a child before all of these things make sense. We are using hindsight today. Where is our foresight?

Things are becoming serious. Because they are becoming bleak, I believe we will be forced to seek a channel of purity.

The advanced iridologist has a message and a philosophy to teach the masses, in spite of the fact that he is working with just a few at the present time. People need to know that drugs and toxins are destroying our world. It's like a little drop of poison oak. As it hits one part of the body, it travels to all areas of the body when it's rubbed or put under hot water. It spreads like wild fire. We've got drug problems spreading like poison throughout humanity today. This can only be taken care of if we take a preventive approach. Remedial programs are not working well.

The iris is the window to good living, or it is the window that reveals a bad way of life. Our living habits, our lifestyle, our food and drug history are all seen through the window of the body, the iris of the eye.

CHAPTER 4
The Scope of Iridology

Iridology deals with analysis, not diagnosis. Diagnosis identifies or determines a disease by means of examination. In contrast, an analysis is the breaking down of a whole into its parts, so that both the parts and the whole can be better understood. Just as a diagnosis is often assisted by x-rays, lab tests, Nuclear Magnetic Resonance imaging, and Electromagnetic Interference scans, an iridology analysis may be of great value in arriving at a diagnosis. Iridology shows things that most diagnostic aids cannot discern.

WHAT IRIDOLOGY CAN DO

Iridology deals with a reflex representation of the activity levels of the various organs of the body, projected into the iris fibers by nerves receiving information from the thalamus and hypothalamus of the brain. The thalamus and hypothalamus are central "relay stations" in the brain, receiving information from every organ, gland, and tissue in the body and passing it along to the iris. In turn, the iris is "mapped out" in such a way that each part of its "geography" represents a specific part of the body. The relative colors of parts of the iris show whether an organ is normal, acute, subacute, chronic, or degenerative in its tissue activity level.

What we see in the iris are signs that indicate stages of inflammation. We also see inherent weaknesses, drug deposits, reflex effects of one organ on another, and mechanical processes such as prolapsus of the transverse colon and diverticula.

That is, we observe the "raw conditions" internal to the body that contribute to a disease, and this information is sufficient for us to develop a treatment program that will work toward correction. The iris is a more reliable indication of what is wrong and where it is wrong in the body than any description of symptoms or set of laboratory tests. This information is enough so that we can intervene nutritionally, through chiropractic, osteopathic, shiatsu, acupuncture, massage, and other therapies.

Often iridology shows "preclinical" signs of problems in an organ, before any actual physical symptoms have appeared. If the correct treatment is promptly given, the problem is corrected before it can manifest into pain, discomfort, or other symptoms. I don't know of any other test or analysis that can do this.

Iridology Can Locate Inflammation

The iridologist concentrates on locating inflammation. Whenever physical signs of inflammation appear (such as fever), the medical doctor cannot tell from these symptoms where the problem is in the body or whether it involves an inherent weakness. Iridology is a master science that can show whether the inflammation involves an inherent weakness, and can give the location of that inflammation.

Iridology Can Identify Tissue Integrity

The iridologist can identify the constitutional background of not only the inflamed tissue, but of every tissue that gives us a reflex reading.

For this reason, we start out knowing that we can determine the integrity of tissue from the standpoint of inflammation. Inflammation always settles in an inherent weakness.

Iridology Can Locate Toxic Material

Through an examination of the iris, we can tell whether toxic material is in an organ. Even if you eat pure foods and drink pure water, you can get toxic material from environmental pollutants and your own metabolic wastes building up in the tissues. Pollution exists in our own body, all the way from an excess of metabolic acids, to gases that we can't expel, and air pollutants and drug residues that we can't eliminate. The fact that we have these settlements in the body is telling us that we have abused the body. These are accumulations that should have no place in our bodies.

Iridology Can Locate Mineral Deficiencies

Another important aspect of iridology is that it allows us to see the mineral deficiencies in specific organs and tissues. When we see an accumulation of toxic material in any organ, we know it cannot function as it should, and it cannot improve its function because of a lack of sufficient mineral assimilation and retention.

Toxic settlements and mineral deficiencies are always found together. When our inherently weak organs do not have enough minerals, the tissue will not function well enough to throw off toxins.

When toxic settlements and mineral deficiencies are found in inherently weak organs, there is a lowering of function. The consequences of lowering of function are inflammation, underactivity, toxic settlement, and mineral deficiency. The identification of these consequences is the main goal of the iridologist.

Iridology Can Show the Need to Replace Old Tissue With New

The iridologist knows that to get rid of any toxic settlement in the body, an elimination must take place, and that this elimination cannot take place until the proper chemical structure exists in the organs. The slightest improvement in the mineral density in any tissue allows the tissue to eliminate toxic settlements, then replace the old, damaged tissue with new. This is called a reversal process.

Iridology Can Reveal a Need for the Reversal Process

This reversal process can be seen in an examination of the iris. This is comparable to taking a laboratory test and finding out that you have less uric acid, the proper rate of creatinine clearance, and other signs of improvement. The reversal process is brought on when healing is taking place, and healing is brought on by replacement, through nutrition, of those chemicals our organs need. We can tell if the tissue is getting well using the therapy that is indicated.

Iridology Can Use Nutrition to Treat Mineral Deficiencies

Most doctors have received only fifteen to twenty hours of instruction in nutrition. They don't know enough about the subject to see how a proper food regimen is necessary to build healthy tissue. Unhealthy tissue must be replaced with tissue that is healthy. When this is accomplished, we actually see our ills leave and new tissue come into its place.

If we knew in advance what the inherent weaknesses were in the body, we could prevent mineral deficiencies and toxic settlements. In fact, iridology is the only analysis that can show us where our inherent weaknesses are, and once we identify those weaknesses, we can develop a program of treatment. This program will include nutrition, climate and exercise, and philosophy. By philosophy, I mean the way we respond to our job, exercise, and marriage—to our whole way of life.

It is even possible for the iridologist to evaluate the positive and negative nutritional needs of the body. The ancient Chinese system of yin and yang is beneficial in determining whether the body is in need of positive mineralization, positive climate, and so forth.

Iridology Can Use Herbs to Treat Chemical Deficiencies

The iridologist often treats these deficiencies with herbs. Herbs have various effects on the different tissues of the body and can be a wonderful help in taking care of mineral deficiencies. In most cases, they are not detrimental to the body, and, best of all, they have no side effects. That is something that cannot be said about drugs!

Iridology Can Monitor Elimination Channel Health

Through an examination of the iris, the iridologist can see ballooned or spastic conditions of the bowel, nerve tension, and stress and strain on the bowel. He can see the digestive capability of the intestinal tract. He can see if the stomach has the proper amount of hydrochloric acid for digestion, and whether there is adequate acidophilus bacteria in the bowel. The iridologist can determine whether the bowel has enough friendly bacteria to keep the electrolytic processes balanced. Crude drug settlements are sometimes seen in the bowel and digestive systems.

The transit time of the bowel can be determined, and the iridologist can tell if the daily bowel movements are three or four days late, being held up in a constipated bowel. Diverticula that are developing in the bowel because of a lack of fiber can be detected. By feeding the bowel properly, beneficial changes can be made.

The iridologist is also able to see prolapsus of the transverse colon, and can observe evidence of pressure from the prolapsus on the organs of the pelvis. He can see evidence of relief after putting the colon back in place.

The iridologist can also monitor the other elimination channels, which are the lungs, the skin, and the kidneys. He can identify the level of function of these organs. Through the cleansing process, the iridologist can bring these organs to their peak level of function.

Iridology Can Locate Nerve Depletion

Nerve depletion can be determined from the iris. This is something that is very difficult for most doctors to find. They usually have to wait until the patient has a nervous breakdown before they realize something is wrong. Sometimes, they have to wait until people are mentally deranged before they can help them. These patients end up at the bottom of a cliff when their fall could—and should—have been prevented.

Iridology Can Monitor the Lymph System

The lymph system flows throughout the whole body, and the iridologist has a wonderful way of monitoring this system. He can tell if it is congested. The murky eye, the "dishwater" eye, and the scurf rim are all indications that the lymph system is dysfunctional. This system holds the key to our immunity. The iridologist can do a great job in helping a person improve his immunity.

Iridology Can Monitor the Brain

The result of physical and mental stress, or fatigue on the body, can be seen by the iridologist. He knows the different brain areas, and that there are lifestyles that are detrimental to certain brain centers. The iridologist can tell his patient what minerals are necessary to build up certain brain faculties.

Potential problems that will contribute to senility can be seen by the iridologist. He can tell when brain faculties are lessened through diminished blood supply to the brain, bringing on lack of memory, lack of comprehension, and lack of mental alertness.

The Iridologist Can Tell the Difference
Between a Healing Crisis and a Disease Crisis

The iridologist can tell the difference between a healing crisis and a disease crisis. As the disease crisis comes on, the patient's symptoms steadily worsen. Sometimes, the patient will die. A healing crisis appears suddenly, after a peak period of good health, and lasts about three days. No one dies in a healing crisis, although nausea, vomiting, fever, diarrhea, and other elimination and symptoms make the patient's condition seem serious. The healing crisis and elimination are nature's way of healing.

One law is followed in the healing crisis: Hering's Law of Cure. Hering's law says, "All disease is cured from within out, from the head down and in reverse order as symptoms were produced in the body." The iris will show when a healing crisis will take place, because the inherent weakness takes on the white color of the acute, overactive stage.

Iridology Can Identify Iatrogenic Disease

The iridologist can see the effect of iatrogenic disease in patterns in the iris. Iatrogenic diseases are diseases that have been caused by drugs that were prescribed to treat a condition. The effects of this disease may have been inherited from past generations, and show up as miasms. A miasm usually indicates that drugs have been used to suppress symptoms.

WHAT IRIDOLOGY CANNOT DO

Although iridology is an excellent tool for identifying many conditions in the body, there are some things it cannot do.

Iridology Cannot See Disease

Specific disease cannot be identified, but indications of tissue inflammation that indicate the presence of some sort of disease or serious problem can be seen. For example, if I find black lesions in the lung area of a person's iris, the condition could be emphysema, tuberculosis, cancer, or some other degenerative disease, but there is no way yet to tell which one it is. It is not necessary for the iridologist to know what the disease is in order to take care of the nutritional needs of the organ with the problem. Iridology is used to find the inflammation and reveal what stage it is in.

Iridology Cannot Predict Blood Pressure

Iridology cannot predict the blood pressure of a person. However, the iridologist knows that people who use a lot of red meat and dairy products tend to be at the high end of the blood pressure scale, while vegetarians tend to be at low normal.

Iridology Cannot Identify What Drugs Are in the Body

Those who practice iridology cannot identify the drugs a person is taking at the present time. Drug deposits such as sulphur and iodine can be seen. These are the two drug categories that are most easily identified. Iron can usually be seen quite easily. It often settles in the bowel and it is one of the things that causes constipation and digestion problems.

Iridology Cannot Discern a Patient's Diet

Iridology cannot tell what diet or foods a person is eating, but can tell when the diet has been imbalanced or inadequate in terms of chemical elements. The iridologist can't say that hot dogs are the cause of a patient's arthritis, or that mince pie is the cause of gout. Common sense tells us that junk food doesn't belong in the body, and iridology can prove it over a period of time by seeing the evidence of increased tissue underactivity.

Iridology Cannot Identify the Surgery a Patient Has Had

The iridologist cannot tell the surgical operations a person has had. The average person who comes into my office has had a tonsillectomy. Many have had an appendectomy. The third most common type of surgery is that of the breast, ovaries, uterus, or gallbladder. All of those conditions developed from acute inflammation, along with the gradual deterioration of the immune system and lymphatic tissues. Chronic disease is developed through suppression. Instead of suppressing the symptoms with drugs, the problem should be treated with foods that nourish the chemical deficiency in the weak organs.

Iridology Cannot Reveal Many Physical Injuries

Many physical injuries leave indications on the iris. Often, however, the injuries are overlooked. It is difficult for the iridologist to tell what injuries have been received from an accident. However, I think if we had more opportunities to examine the eyes of people who have had auto accidents and other physical accidents, I believe we'd be able to document iris changes.

The iridologist cannot tell if a snake has bitten a person, or if a person has been recently poisoned. He can't tell the cause of a coma, or what to do about it.

Iridology Cannot Identify the Kinds of Toxins in the Body

Those who practice iridology cannot identify the kind of toxic settlement that is in the body, or just what elements comprise that settlement. We can only tell there is a toxic deposit in a certain tissue. This deposit could be catarrh, metabolic acids, heavy metals, drug residues, or a combination of several or all of them.

Iridology Cannot Determine a Person's Hormone Level

Hormone levels don't show up in the iris. It is impossible for the iridologist to tell if someone is using birth control pills, nor is pregnancy evident in the iris, at least at the present time; the day may come when the iridologist can tell whether a woman is pregnant and what gender the child will be.

Iridology Cannot Reveal Sexually Transmitted Disease

One of the greatest weaknesses of iridology, I feel, is that the iridologist cannot identify sexually transmitted disease. I know AIDS is one of the worst scourges that has come upon humanity, but the iridologist cannot tell from the iris whether the AIDS virus is attacking leukocytes.

LET'S BE FAIR IN EVALUATING HEALTH ARTS

There are failures in the medical profession and there are failures in the drugless profession. Those who use iridology have had failures. If it were 100 percent sure, I am certain every newspaper would write about it. Often, the media are only too eager to report mistakes. If you want to get publicity, make a mistake! However, I feel each health art should be judged by its success and what it has to offer. Drugs and surgery have their place in extreme situations where less invasive methods are not appropriate or have not worked, but nutrition, chiropractic, osteopathic, homeopathy, acupuncture, and other drugless arts should be tried before we resort to drugs or surgery. Keep in mind that no tissue correction, no true healing, can take place without proper nutrition to supply the chemical elements needed.

Drugs cannot build new tissue, nor can homeopathic remedies. The health arts involving mechanical adjustments cannot build new tissue, and their effectiveness depends on nutritional support. Iridology can, in all cases, be used to monitor the rate of healing and the rate at which any therapy or program is bringing correction to tissue.

Diagnosis and treatment are changing every day. The medical doctor is beginning to look for signs he never looked for before. He is looking at infrared photography of the body, sonograms, Nuclear Magnetic Resonance, and EMI scans. Diagnostic approaches are changing.

Western medicine does not have a 100 percent record in its diagnoses, which is why doctors still use exploratory surgery to look inside patients and try to figure out what is wrong, and why people get second opinions from other doctors. There are mistakes in prescriptions and treatments. This places Western medicine in the category of a health art, rather than an exact science.

IRIDOLOGY REQUIRES FURTHER EXPLORATION

There is still so much unexplored territory in the field of iridology. At the present time there is much we can determine from an analysis of the iris, but there is so much more that we do not know. It is time for all those interested in combining iridology and nutrition to come together and begin exploring this exciting field!

CHAPTER 5
A New Breed of Doctor

Recently, a magazine writer sat through a series of my talks. After the lecture, she asked, "Where are the doctors for this new approach to health care you've been talking about?"

This new profession of doctors is not yet in existence. Or, if it exists, it is in embryo form—growing, developing, and receiving nourishment from the ideas and experiences of thousands of men and women in many health arts who are finding out how to get healthy and stay healthy in a world where disease, not health, is the norm. The new profession is yet to be born.

Presently, we are taught to go to the doctor when we have symptoms. That may be too late. The disease may have already progressed to the point of malignancy.

The dictionary defines malignant as, "Evil in nature . . . extremely malevolent or malicious . . . tending to produce death or deterioration . . . to infiltrate, metastasize and terminate fatally." Malignancy is bad news. We primarily identify it with cancer, and when we go to the doctor with cancer symptoms, it is usually too late.

The great need of the average citizen of planet Earth is to know how to live a healthy, productive life, free from disease. Today, very few doctors practice preventive health care, but I would not advise going to any other kind. The doctor who is interested in keeping you well is of infinitely greater value than the doctor who says he can't do anything until you are sick.

What kind of profession is it that thrives and grows wealthy on sickness and disease, but shows so little interest in maintaining health? Somehow, rightful priorities have turned topsy-turvy.

My late friend, Dr. Alan Nittler, once wrote a book titled *A New Breed of Doctor*, in which he discussed the tremendous role nutrition will play in the therapeutic approach of doctors of the future. Dr. Nittler was speaking from personal experience—he used the wholistic healing art in his practice and knew the healing properties of foods. The future doctor will be like Dr. Nittler, aware of all the healing techniques and approaches. He will be able to select exactly the right program or therapy for each patient.

Medical practice is becoming increasingly depersonalized and drug oriented. Norman Cousins, former editor of *Saturday Review*, has suggested that America is on the verge of becoming a nation of hypochondriacs, partly because of massive exposure to television and magazine ads that push medication and urge people to "see your doctor if symptoms persist." Most doctors are now incorporated, either individually or through a clinic or partnership. There are no more home visits, and free treatment of the poor is almost unheard of. This, obviously, is far from even the doctor of the past, the compassionate professional who took care of all who needed help. Now it is time for a new breed of doctor!

At a convention of the American Medical Association in Las Vegas, Nevada, 120 doctors took a simple ten-question quiz on nutrition designed by Dr. Michael Latham of Cornell University. More than 90 percent failed the test. "Judging by their answers to these ten question," said Dr. Latham, "very few could be expected to give sound nutritional advice to their patients." The new kind of doctor must know all about nutrition.

Because of rising dissatisfaction with conventional Western medicine, doctors have taken a big drop in popularity. A recent Harris Poll showed that people who had "a great deal of confidence in medicine" dropped from 73 percent in 1966 to 32 percent in 1982. I believe this is a sign that the American people are beginning to wake up to the need for a new breed of doctor.

Most physical examinations today are very crude and not particularly revealing to the doctors who make them. Laboratory tests are often ambiguous and inconclusive. Diagnoses are often tentative, founded on very little solid evidence, and incomplete. They seldom offer much of a profile of what is going on in the whole body, particularly if drugs are being taken.

Iridology analyses, in my view, offer much more information about the state of the body than do the examinations of Western medicine, and I feel they are much more reliable. Because of this, I believe the new breed of doctor will want to know iridology.

WHO WILL BE THE PATIENTS?

Most people are accustomed to present-day medicine, and dependent upon drugs, surgery, and the idea of the "quick cure." It will be difficult to persuade these people to go to a doctor who works with nature and not against it.

A doctor, no matter how brilliant, well-trained, and wise in the ways of healing, is no doctor at all without patients. The new-day doctors are going to have to touch a responsive chord in people to persuade them to try the "new approach." It will take a good deal of education before we will see this change.

People used to demanding "instant" results from powerful prescription drugs are going to have to learn that nature's way is slow, but sure. Drugs don't heal anything; they block symptoms. People are going to learn that they must change their lifestyle before they will see changes in their body. Until they are willing to follow the teaching of the new-day doctor, nothing will change. No true healing will take place. We need to see a new breed of patient.

CONTEMPORARY HEALTH PROBLEMS

The new breed of doctor must be aware of the health problems of people today. People are wearing nylon and polyester clothes, walking on rubber-soled shoes, wearing glasses that cut out 95 percent of the ultraviolet light, watching color televisions that emit radiation, and cooking food in microwave ovens. Every home has at least a half-dozen electrical appliances. In many ways, we have changed or increased our exposure to electromagnetic vibrations without knowing how they affect our bodies. We can be certain of one thing—these finer forces do, in fact, affect us.

Many people work under fluorescent lights, around high levels of noise, and in buildings where chemical fumes rise from the rugs, office equipment, and drapes, and are breathed along with the air. There seem to be harsh colors that increase the level of accidents in factories and soft colors that reduce it. These are things that most people—including doctors—are not aware of, and they affect us emotionally and physically.

Most Americans are aware that health problems are increasing, and that present-day doctors seem unable to stem the tide. We are coming to the place where people will realize that there must be a change—there must be a new way.

Cancer continues to claim thousands of lives each year, despite the fact that billions of dollars have been spent over the past several decades to find a cure for it. How much time and money have been spent on prevention? According to the American Cancer Society, it takes twenty years or so for some types of cancer to develop. Where was the doctor twenty years ago? One cancer, one major heart operation, one severe chronic disease can wipe out a lifetime of savings. Where are the doctors who can help us stay healthy and avoid all this unnecessary suffering?

How many patients are ready to take the time and make the effort to get well? How many patients want to continue to live in the dark ages, thinking that doctors can cure, that doctors understand the mysteries of life, that doctors have a secret that is going to get them well? People want to get well overnight; they want a magic pill. How many patients know that it takes time for the body to make changes? To make the proper tissue changes, you have to have a doctor who knows how to work with the body, and he can work only as fast as the body works.

THE BODY IS LIKE A MACHINE

It is not a matter of stimulation or sedation. It is not a matter of tranquilizing the body and finding ways to bring one organ back to health without involving the rest of the body. The body works as a whole organism. It is something like a machine that works according to a definite plan, and we have to get back to this God-created plan to know how to operate it. We don't go out and buy oil for our joints or hinges; we don't go out and buy a new valve; we are trying to treat the body like a machine, but we still haven't learned how to use and care for it. Most of us have problems like that of a carbon-clogged exhaust muffler, unable to get rid of toxic fuel wastes. Our elimination is very poor. Usually, this is because our eating habits are very poor. We don't know how to treat this machine.

Have you ever tried putting the body's chassis up on a shelf for a couple of days to give it a rest? Have you had a checkup lately? Do you know what kind of checkup you need? Do you have the right fuel—the right chemical elements? How many patients know that they need calcium when they have bone trouble? That phosphorus is needed when the brain has become slow and unresponsive? That lecithin is necessary for a good memory and concentration? Most people don't know these things, so in the future, we must educate the patient. Then, we will have a new breed of patient.

THE PATIENT MUST WORK WITH THE DOCTOR

It is when the doctor and the patient work as one, in agreement, that there will be true healing. Getting rid of a pain or two so the patient thinks he is getting better is not real healing.

The doctor who is going to lead the way in the future is one with a higher consciousness. He will be interested in the soul growth of his patients. He will be interested in seeing that they have the best there is from the soil, the best from the sea, and the best the sun can produce. He will know about the living habits of his patients; he will tell them what foods they should eat, and will see that their elimination channels are working properly. The new kind of patient will listen to the doctor and follow his instructions.

The new-day doctor will have the proper training and education to lead the patient on this new path. Unless he gets that path straightened out, the doctor and the patient will remain as far apart as they are today.

These days, we don't even know what kind of doctor to seek out for a particular problem. We seek chiropractic help when we need nutrition. We take a doctor "on faith" because he says he can help us. A doctor should never tell a patient he can help him unless he means it. Disappointment breeds doubt, doubt breeds cynicism, and cynicism breeds dis-ease.

If a patient's symptoms indicate a need for chiropractic therapy and the doctor can't take care of the problem, he should refer the patient to someone who can. The patient should be sent to a doctor who will teach him as well as treat him. The new breed of doctor should be more interested in keeping his patients well and happy than in treating them for ailments and diseases. He should be interested in preventing disease. He should recognize how wonderfully we are made, that our body is a "loaned instrument," and that we must take care of it.

PEOPLE SHOULD BE TAUGHT HOW TO STAY HEALTHY

A new orientation in health care will come to our schools, one that will emphasize prevention of disease. People will find that there are many things that hinder health mentally, physically, and spiritually, and we will have to become aware of these things. But, until we have a new breed of doctor, the kind of doctor who can recognize that the patient must be involved in the therapeutic process, we will not see a complete healing.

When this does happen, it will raise patient confidence and consciousness and will raise our educational consciousness. We will develop institutions to promote health instead of institutions to fight disease and sickness. People will learn how to build and maintain health and high-level well-being.

Now, doctors are seeing "waiting room" patients. The new doctor will be interested in checkups to see that patients are perfectly well, that they have all the chemical elements they need, and that problems are taken care of before symptoms develop. He is going to take care of his patients ahead of time.

IT'S TIME FOR A CHANGE

The doctor of the future will influence the political process and the food and drug laws. He will see that restaurants do not serve food that brings on degeneration. He will have a voice in food processing, manufacturing, and packaging. In the future, we will have hospitals that will not allow patients to check out before they know how to change their habits and prevent future recurrences of their condition. We will learn how to cook right.

Before they marry, couples of the future will know how to take care of themselves, so that the next generation will be stronger and healthier than their parents. There is no reason why we should raise children as future doctor's bills. We need doctors who guide us to make sure we remain in good health, strong, and mentally alert.

The new breed of doctor will have a complete understanding of how all environmental conditions affect the chemistry and physiology of man. He will understand what lighting conditions are needed in our factories and work places, and will know what role sunlight plays in our health. He will know about air quality, radiation, noise, climate, jet lag, and freeway stress—all of the everyday factors that affect human health. He will know how to use color, music, fasting, foods, juices, mechanical therapies, and vibratory processes to restore homeostasis in the body.

Perhaps the new breed of doctor will oversee the development of films that will make people laugh and speed up the healing process, or films that release stress, resentment, and resistance. He may teach breathing exercises that balance left side and right side body energies. Maybe he will teach color visualization exercises to raise the metabolic rate of particular organs.

The most important thing to take care of in man is the soul, and the new breed of doctor and patient must understand that the purpose of the soul is to express and grow. However, this can only be done when both doctor and patient come together to work for the higher values in life, seeking the higher path. Man deserves the best that God has for him.

PART TWO

Disease: The Consequences of an Unnatural Lifestyle

CHAPTER 6
Which Path Are You On?

I try to use constructive principles from nature to help patients get on the pathway to health. These include sunshine, fresh air, pure water, pure foods, proper amount of rest, and moral feelings consistent with the universal principle of life. Sleep, rest, vitality, and energy economy are very important. As we work in this direction, the body is able to strengthen itself, eventually emerging as whole, pure, and clean.

We use constructive principles in nature to improve and repair. Use of these nature principles helps our body do the best it can, according to the potential our genes have made possible from the very beginning.

There are many factors working against us that cause disease. The factors are destructive, not constructive, and often go against nature. Too many people are on this pathway to disease.

FACTORS THAT CONTRIBUTE TO THE BUILDING OF A DISEASE

Destructive principles are habits we become attached to, poor lifestyle and attitude habits that contribute to the deterioration of health. This lifestyle may involve junk foods, drugs, alcohol abuse, impure air, polluted water, and foods that do not have the mineral elements they should have.

Nature has its own way of doing things, and the more we move off the path of what I call "the nature cure principles," the more we develop disease, symptoms, pains, and aches. Sometimes, we wonder how these problems can develop in a natural body that God has created. We realize that there are not only creative principles working in the human body, but creative principles working in our environment, in our foods, and in our emotions. This is nature's way, a harmonious way of living and a harmonious way to build the best of health. The best of health comes when the mental, moral, and spiritual levels conform to the best that nature can provide for the well-being of human life.

Many times, disease can be considered a result of inharmonious activity existing within our body. The electromagnetic activity is not right. The electrolytes are not working well with each other. There are mineral deficiencies and chemical imbalances. There is a destructive principle that takes place when there is disharmony in the body, and the eventual result is disease.

It is not easy to know all the factors that produce destruction in the body. But if we know what nature's laws are, we can conform to them. When there is a violation of natural law, disease develops in the body.

When natural law is violated, the vital spirit is not working in all the organs, and vitality is lowered. The body cannot rebuild and rejuvenate. There are toxic settlements in the various elimination organs. These must be tended to so we can be clean and pure within.

In a diseased body, there is abnormal composition of blood and lymph. The blood lacks the material to build and repair. The lymph may be low in the immunity factors that usually protect us from the disease that surrounds us. The blood and lymph can only become clean and normal when our elimination organs are clean and normal.

There are inherent weaknesses in organs, glands, and tissues where morbid materials, poisons, drug residues, and metabolic wastes can settle. We need to know which organs, glands, and tissues have these inherent weaknesses. When we take care of our inherent weaknesses, we start to rebuild our body and prevent disease.

Any of the previously mentioned factors will hinder and inhibit normal function in the body. Any of these lowers the energies in the body. The vibratory rates begin to drop into a lower harmonic scale. Good health cannot come and stay when we are at this level.

The body follows a pathway in life. Because of this, there is really no way we can say there is a "cure" for any disease. It is when we are off the path of good health that we find disease comes automatically into a body, developing and evolving of its own accord.

There are four levels of inflammation in all the diseases we develop, and each one represents a progressively worsened condition. These four levels are acute, subacute, chronic, and degenerative. These stages are presented in Figure 6.1. This figure illustrates the correlation between the natural light of the iris and good health versus the darkness of the iris in proportion to the degree of degeneration in the body.

THE ACUTE STAGE OF DISEASE

The acute level of inflammation occurs when nature tries to throw off and eliminate from the body the waste that is associated with the inflammation. Waste is eliminated in the form of catarrh, phlegm and mucus, acid discharges, foreign matter, and toxins. When the body is doing this, it is called a "cleansing process." In most cases, this cleansing process should never be interfered with.

It is in this acute stage of activity in the body and the natural elimination that is taking place that the body is restored to health. We should never stop a catarrhal elimination for this reason. My job, as iridologist, is to promote and supervise this natural elimination. If toxins are not allowed to be eliminated, the patient will progress into what is called the "subacute stage."

THE SUBACUTE STAGE

The subacute stage develops whenever we use drugs as a suppressive measure to drive catarrhal discharges back into the body. When toxic material is driven back into the body it lodges in various organs and tissues, producing pain, fever, aches, and discomfort. These symptoms are a warning to take care of this subacute condition. If it is not taken care of, disease conditions will worsen.

We can almost consider the acute condition as a healing crisis. It is an elimination process. If we let the elimination happen, the body will return to its natural healthy state and the subacute stage will be avoided. Catarrhal eliminations that are suppressed in the acute stage are the beginnings of disease.

It is through the study of iridology that we find out most clearly how a disease is built and how it is reversed. A disease is "undone" by going back over the path or track on which it was built. The healing crisis can be reached naturally by following a right way of living.

THE CHRONIC STAGE OF DISEASE

The chronic stage of inflammation is a further development of underactivity following the subacute stage of a disease. In this stage, healing agents are forced to "take a back seat."

When we overpower all of the natural defenses of the body with drugs, chemicals from polluted air and water, undesirable foods, and other processes of a destructive nature, Nature can no longer do her duty. There is a certain amount of vitality that goes along with good health and when that vitality is lost, chronic disease comes upon us.

Chronic diseases are made. We eat and drink them into existence. We think them into existence. We have emotional problems, work problems, marriage problems, and people problems. All of these problems waste our vitality. In the end, our body no longer has the power or energy to overcome disease.

A chronic disease is really a condition in which one or more organs is unable to react and eliminate properly. The organ is so underactive that it is unable to rid itself of toxins or rebuild damaged tissue. The constitutional strength of the body is being overcome.

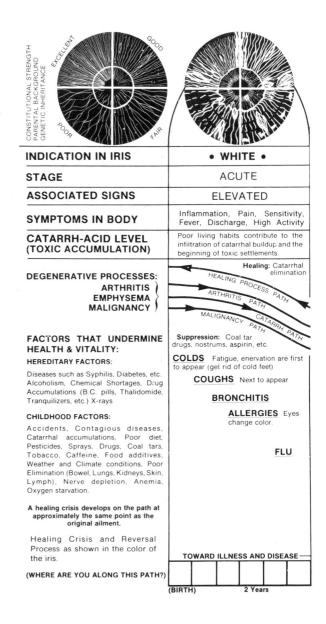

Figure 6.1   Pathways to Health and Disease
Observed in the Iris of the Eye

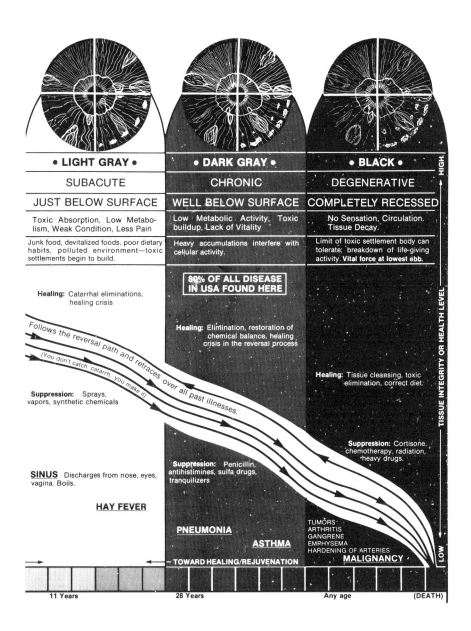

• **LIGHT GRAY** •	• **DARK GRAY** •	• **BLACK** •	HIGH
SUBACUTE	CHRONIC	DEGENERATIVE	
JUST BELOW SURFACE	WELL BELOW SURFACE	COMPLETELY RECESSED	
Toxic Absorption, Low Metabolism, Weak Condition, Less Pain	Low Metabolic Activity, Toxic buildup, Lack of Vitality	No Sensation, Circulation. Tissue Decay.	
Junk food, devitalized foods, poor dietary habits, polluted environment—toxic settlements begin to build.	Heavy accumulations interfere with cellular activity.	Limit of toxic settlement body can tolerate; breakdown of life-giving activity. **Vital force at lowest ebb.**	

80% OF ALL DISEASE IN USA FOUND HERE

Healing: Catarrhal eliminations, healing crisis

Healing: Elimination, restoration of chemical balance, healing crisis in the reversal process

Healing: Tissue cleansing, toxic elimination, correct diet.

Follows the reversal path and retraces over all past illnesses. (You don't catch catarrh, you make it)

Suppression: Sprays, vapors, synthetic chemicals

Suppression: Cortisone, chemotherapy, radiation, heavy drugs.

Suppression: Penicillin, antihistimines, sulfa drugs, tranquilizers

SINUS Discharges from nose, eyes, vagina. Boils.

HAY FEVER

PNEUMONIA

ASTHMA

TUMORS
ARTHRITIS
GANGRENE
EMRHYSEMA
HARDENING OF ARTERIES
MALIGNANCY

→ TOWARD HEALING/REJUVENATION ←

TISSUE INTEGRITY OR HEALTH LEVEL

LOW

| 11 Years | 28 Years | Any age | (DEATH) |

THE DEGENERATIVE STAGE

The degenerative, or final stage of a disease, is characterized by almost total loss of function in an organ or tissue area. In most cases, nothing can be done to reverse a condition that has developed this far. Tissue destruction is too great, and the body's immune system is unable to respond. Overall, the body is too weak for other organs and systems to be strengthened and uplifted so they can help the degenerative organ or tissue recover. I don't want to say reversal cannot take place at this stage, because I've seen it happen. However, it is very rare. Many times the patient is too weak to bring to a healing crisis, which is his only hope.

When we have allowed disease-building processes to remain in our lives, we earn the consequences that go with these processes. Some people are aware that many of their habits are self-destructive, but they are not willing to change. At the degenerative stage of disease, the great majority have bought their tickets to the other side, and there are seldom any return tickets.

THE HEALING CRISIS

The healing crisis is an acute reaction that naturally comes when the body has the energy to throw off toxic materials. It results from ascendancy of nature's healing forces over disease conditions. When the inflamed organs have been identified and a diet containing the proper nutrients is followed, the body gains strength and is ready to perform its own cure in its own way. The healing crisis is the best way to cooperate with nature and see her fullest glory. Nature will bring us back to the health we are supposed to have.

The healing crisis tells us that we are working toward recovery. It works with nature's constructive principles and Hering's law of cure: "All disease is cured from within out, from the head down, and in reverse order as symptoms have appeared in the body."

When we in iridology look at the development of a disease, we start by noticing the acute signs in the iris, going into the darker subacute signs, where elimination processes are set aside and the body is using all of its energy just to get by. To put it literally, we are just existing, just crawling through life. We cannot say we feel wonderful and really mean it.

The healing crisis has some features in common with a disease crisis, but it is the *reversal* of the disease. Disease crises are not the same as healing crises. Healing crises occur at times when we feel at the peak of good health, and they last only three days or so.

The disease crisis is a reaction resulting from an ascendancy of disease conditions over the healing forces of the organism. There is a fight going on. It is only in the reversal process, when the body goes back over the inflammation and symptoms of the past, that we can come to the healing crisis. Most disease crises have a fatal termination.

THE PATHWAY TO HEALTH

There are methods to follow in order to stay in good health. We should establish uplifting surroundings. We need an environment we are comfortable in. We need to have the proper occupation, marry the right person, and have friends around us to give us the emotional balance we should have. We should have the proper food and chemical balance in the body. Our bodies should be toxin-free. It should be a great privilege for us to live according to the laws of nature in order to have the healthiest body possible.

The body should have exercise every day. We must build up the blood naturally, by eating the right foods in the right proportions. We should recognize that cleanliness is important through eliminating the waste matter in our body, and that oxygenation is necessary to build up the thyroid gland.

There are special bowel cleansing methods, such as colonics and colemas, that can take away an excessive amount of toxic material that has settled there over a long period of time. We need to promote the elimination of this waste matter.

We must account for our own health. We are here to take care of this body in the best way possible, so we should seek out the best teaching. We should seek out beauty, exercise, care, and concern for our appearance to motivate us to stay in as fit a condition as possible.

Can We Use Drugs?

A question many people ask is: "Can drugs be used in conformity with the constructive principle of nature?"

I acknowledge that there are some things that drugs can do. First of all, they can do everything they claim to do. They can hold in abatement any pain, ache, or discharge, and they can make symptoms disappear. However, drugs do not enter into developing a well-nourished tissue structure. No tissue can use drugs nutritionally, and only nutrition can restore damaged tissue.

When treating chronic problems, it is best not to be using drugs at first, but to try more natural methods to bring on a reversal or healing crisis. This reversal process, or acute stage, will bring on the good health most people are seeking. Drugs do not bring about a healing crisis.

Drugs produce side effects. Drug residues may settle in the body and produce genetic changes, interfering with the next generation, often reducing resistance to disease.

Drugs can have time-bomb effects. In many cases, we do not foresee what consequences will develop from using drugs. Drug residues in tissue cause psora, miasms, and medeic conditions that do not emerge until years later in chronic and degenerative disease. Side effects become part of the tissue. The tissues cannot work, perform, or function normally.

Drugs can suppress any symptom, ache, or discharge in our body, driving an acute stage inflammation into a subacute and underactive tissue stage, where toxic materials are driven back into the body. This is the beginning of the many chronic diseases we have today.

Drugs produce temporary relief. They are not corrective, because they don't make new tissue in place of the old. Drugs do not conform to the replacement therapy idea of putting new tissue in place of old.

Of course, not everyone wants the best. Many people are not interested in having a new body. They are not interested in replacement therapy. They live on excuses, blaming God, nature, people, or the environment, rather than straightening out their lives and living the natural life that would give them the best health possible.

There are times when I believe drugs are necessary, but those times are rare. When a headache gets too big, we take "triple-strength" pain killers. We are not only taking one kind of aspirin, but aspirin plus other compounds. Cough syrups have a suppressive effect that stops the elimination that should be taking place. These toxic materials then back up in the various systems of our body, creating conditions for a future disease. All diseases that come upon man in the form of a deranged natural or organic human function can be stopped with drugs, but it is better, in most cases, to allow a natural elimination to take place, and not develop a more chronic condition.

Natural Remedies

There are many elementary remedies to consider. Homeopathic remedies have healing properties, as do water, air, light, magnetism, electricity, and climatic conditions. Altitude can also be considered as a means of healing.

There are other remedies, such as scientific food selections or combinations that use various vitamins, enzymes, and mineral supplements. We may need to take care of chemical deficiencies, balancing the chemical elements in our body. To do this, an awareness of herbs, natural extracts, and the vital chemical remedies that are available to us through fruits, vegetables, flowers, nuts, and seeds is necessary. Mechanical remedies such as polarity therapy, shiatsu, and reflex therapies may help. There may even be times when surgery has to be considered, but any time surgery can be avoided, I believe it should be. It should not be the first choice in taking care of a problem.

We often underrate mental and spiritual remedies. This is not a matter of religion—it is a matter of spiritual principle. It means following that which God is directing us to do, and finding out what is right, not who is right. It is not a matter of living up to society and what it can do for you, but what you can do for yourself. This way of living brings a good feeling and a natural way of life.

HOW ACUTE DISEASES ARE ACQUIRED

Acute diseases usually begin when we are infants. Infants inherit inherent weaknesses in organs from their parents. In many cases, the weaknesses are accompanied by lowered resistance to disease.

In the beginning of life, the child has acute catarrhal diseases. Then he proceeds through the various stages when drug encumbrances develop through infantile diseases and suppression of catarrhal conditions. Finally, the child develops underactivity in the inherently weak organs.

Encumbrances may be passed down from the parents, or problems may come from pregnant mothers who aren't living correctly. A good deal of this can be eliminated through proper living in the early years. If the infant is placed in the right conditions, and shown how to live in harmony with the laws of nature, the child will be healthy.

At an early age of life we should learn to develop a natural immunity. The natural laws should work well in every organ in the body. If we do not see that this takes place, secondary causes come in. Germs, parasites, skin eruptions, catarrhal discharges of all kinds, ulcers, and so forth begin to develop. This is nature's way of trying to bring itself back to normal.

Many people assume that bacteria are the primary cause of most disease. However, bacteria are a secondary condition. The whole body is the most important thing to consider. Otherwise, bacterial diseases are treated by killing the bacteria, with drugs that may harm the body in other ways. These drugs could be antiseptics, serums, vaccines, and antibiotics.

I do not believe that germs cause disease. In most cases, germs cannot live or multiply in a healthy body. They do not assert themselves as disease. Tubercular germs are found in the throats of 90 percent of the population, but that doesn't mean these people have tuberculosis. We consider the microorganisms that can attack the body as the secondary form of disease, that can thrive because there is something in the body for them to feed on. We have to take care of the host first. We have to keep well. We cannot be anemic and we must be clean and vigorous from within. Then, we will not be affected by disease taints and germs from without.

Bacteria are ever-present and all around us. We must take care of the host at all times. We must control harmful microorganisms by not allowing them to gain control of our body. We should use as many of the health procedures as necessary in order to have good health.

TREATING DISEASES NATURALLY

If we raise our children to follow the natural pathway, they will know what to do as they grow older. Health will accompany them through life if they remain on this path. The time to start a natural lifestyle is in infancy.

Dealing With Childhood Illness the Natural Way

In the beginning of a child's life there will be colds, coughs, fevers, bronchial disturbances, stomach upsets, and vomiting spells. This is nature trying to normalize the child's system, and the time most people start a suppression program.

When a child develops an acute disease of any kind, we should let it run its natural course. The mother must not become impatient and lose faith in natural treatment. It may take a week or more to even cure a common cold in the head or an attack of bronchitis, or from two to eight weeks to cure a case of whooping cough. Serenity, cheerfulness, and patience are the primary requisites of the nature cure physician. The natural treatment is very much the same in all acute inflammatory ailments.

The baby should not be forced to eat, but he should be able to easily handle vegetable and fruit juices. These can be given to him every two to three hours. All of the child's energy will go to the elimination system, rather than the digestive system. In most cases, these things will clear up in a few days.

Try to keep your child on a "preventive program." Don't be tempted to resort to suppressive means of taking care of all the different "itises" that are included in the acute forms of inflammation children can get. Children need proper guidance, and must have the good example of their parents to follow. They should be given the example of prevention, not suppression.

Nearly all children start out in life with acute conditions, such as nasal problems and ear problems. When these problems occur, parents should learn to allow these eliminations to take place. If children are put on a proper feeding program, these discharges can be prevented. Most childhood illnesses are not fatal, and serious problems are created by trying to suppress them. Suppression drives toxic materials back into the body. We should, instead, change our way of living by feeding our children natural, whole foods.

Unfortunately, very few mothers know how to feed children properly. They don't know that the formulas they use are synthetic food, not real food, and may cause diabetic tendencies in later years. We need whole foods to build whole bodies.

After the first year of life, when nature wants to respond to chemical changes in the child's body, the milk they are normally given has to be supplemented with some of the iron foods. Enough iron is held in the liver to meet the needs of the first year of the child's life, but after the first year, the iron that was stored in the liver will be used up, and we must give the child some iron foods. Milk is lacking in iron.

Iron assimilation can be aided by adding natural foods like liquid chlorophyll or blackstrap molasses to the milk. They are both high in iron. Cut out all white sugar and keep the amount of wheat intake low. Follow my program of using the four cereal substitutes for wheat: corn meal, millet, brown rice, and oats.

Carrots, beets, zucchini, banana squash, and all summer squash are wonderful for a baby when he begins to eat solid foods. Don't forget that a baby can be anemic, so make sure he is getting enough iron, folic acid, and vitamin B_{12}.

We should teach our children that elimination is the most important thing to take care of in the body, and the bowel is the most important eliminative organ. They should be taught what foods to eat to care for the bowel.

All yellow foods have a laxative effect. Greens also have a laxative effect. Fruits, vegetables, and whole grains are rich in the fiber we need to give bulk to the stool. Fiber helps shorten bowel transit time, which keeps the bowel clean and reduces the intake of toxins from the bowel to the bloodstream.

Poor elimination develops first in the bowel, second in the bronchial tubes, third in the skin, and fourth in the kidneys. All parents should know about these four channels and teach their children to take care of themselves properly. These organs must be kept toxin-free and chemical deficiencies must be fed. Proof of toxic buildup is seen in the fact that often, by the age of five or six, children develop tonsillitis and have their tonsils removed. The reason tonsils become infected is because of toxic accumulations.

Exercise is important in keeping the elimination organs and the lymph system moving. Children don't usually have to be told that they need exercise. They love to run, jump, crawl under and over things, and climb trees. They seem to get all the exercise they need.

Children have natural, inborn traits. Some are mechanically inclined, some musically inclined. To be happy, people should do some of the things they love to do. A child's life should be happy, but disciplined. We have to teach children that discipline that comes from nature.

Staying on the Natural Path During the Teen Years

As children grow into teenagers, allergies, bronchitis, and flu develop. Other acute conditions that occur are colds, gastritis, skin rash, acne, dandruff, vaginitis, hay fever, headaches, and irritable bowel.

This age is a very dangerous one. Teenagers have observed the habits of their parents for some time, and are becoming more dependent. They begin to develop confidence and to reason and make their own decisions. Mentally, they are getting to the place where they resent the authority of their parents. Many teenagers resist authority, which can result in nerve ring problems or other nerve problems. Iridology shows this. As stubborness and obstinance show up in the teenager's personality, their weaknesses emerge.

Teenagers are making glandular changes. Girls are coming into womanhood and boys into manhood. Between the ages of twelve and fourteen, changes begin in both sexes. When these glandular changes start to take place, there is a change in the personality. These personality changes tend to influence where teenagers like to be and what they like and don't like to do. They begin to try out things when their parents aren't looking.

Parents should not give up trying to teach their children during these years. When parents teach children, it is beneficial to both of them. Parents should see that their children get into good company, because they will find enough bad company on their own. The city streets of today are filled with bad influences. Drug addiction often begins in the teenage years. Moral standards are formed in the teens. It is up to the parents to set the example in moral standards. Parents do their greatest teaching by being the greatest influence.

If you smoke, you can't tell your child not to smoke. If you drink, you can't tell your child not to drink. If you are using drugs, you can't expect your child not to use them. Children find out they have a life of their own. They take on their own responsibilities. They have to experiment. This age is very difficult.

We should show our children how to fit into society and how to get along with others. Parents should spend more time than ever with their children during these years. I have heard that 60 percent of children return to empty homes after school. These children are called "latch-key kids." They are left to themselves, without parental supervision. If a child is left without supervision, he will find a way to get into trouble.

Teenagers should be taught about vibrations, so they will know the value of music, and what music can do to the body. There should be experiments with music to show what rock and roll music will do, as compared with classical music. I believe rock and roll has a detrimental effect upon the body and brain. Teenagers should also know the value of color and what it means to follow a more natural way of life.

There should not be a minority doing this; it should be a majority. During these years, children gain the experience they need to become adults. Everyone wants good judgment. Where do you get that good judgment? From experience. How do you get experience? Through bad judgment. These times of learning occur during the teenage years.

Parents shouldn't allow themselves to be isolated from their children. They can get involved in exercise and sports with their children and should encourage their teenagers to ski, hike, and swim. Through these activities they will learn lessons that will stay with them the rest of their lives.

Our children should be taught how to have healthy bodies. Proper nutrition should not be neglected! It is during these years that they want to eat hot dogs, hamburgers, and sodas.

What a person eats has a lot to do with his mental life and personality. Many mental difficulties can be overcome by a chemically well-balanced body. A healthy mind helps you to better decide what to do for the future. ture.

How the twig is bent determines how the tree will grow. It is up to you to give your child the best you possibly can. A parent of a teenage child faces a great challenge! Parents should be in the best health possible. They should be able to show by experience what is right and what is wrong.

More subacute conditions begin in the teenage years. Constipation may begin during these years, and respiratory troubles may develop. If our teenagers haven't been properly taught, this is where suppression begins. This is the time they learn to use aspirin for headaches and to use laxatives when their bowels are not moving. At this age they develop acne, and begin to treat skin trouble from the outside instead of from within. Practices such as these result in the formation of subacute conditions.

When it comes to elimination, animals and babies have no inhibitions. Teenagers become inhibited and start to develop subacute conditions. All discharges are suppressed, because they interfere with playing time. All of these factors contribute to the development of the disease process.

A Time for Decision

I call the age between twenty and forty the chronic stage. It is then that people suffer for their past lifestyles if they did not stay on the natural path. The effect of our upbringing will show at this age, and it is at this time that we find we have made mistakes. Sometimes, we want to blame our parents: "They should have known better. Why did they give me all that Danish pastry when I was a child? Why did they let me eat all that candy?"

As children, we lived where our parents lived. They probably lived there because their jobs were nearby. Maybe the area we grew up in was polluted, or the climate was damp. Perhaps the climate and air aggravated our inherent weaknesses.

At the young adult stage, we should realize that our children will be as healthy as we are. We must be examples to our children. Now we should rethink our lifestyle and make the decision to follow Nature's way. We may be sorry for not following better health habits earlier in life, but we still have time to change!

If you have developed a chronic disease such as arthritis or asthma, this is the time to seek a reversal. Don't further suppress your symptoms with penicillin, antihistamines, sulphur drugs, or tranquilizers.

Avoiding Illness in Middle Age

Our adult years eventually flow into middle age. This is the time when we want to enjoy success. At this time we're using brain and nerve forces we've never used before. By this age, we should be very aware of our health, and should work toward avoiding chronic disease by learning the best ways to reverse them. We should be working toward keeping the body's energies at the highest peak possible.

I find it astonishing that men and women gain weight after they are married. I don't know if it is because they "let themselves go," or if they have more chronic conditions established in their bodies. At middle age, the thyroid becomes underactive and the metabolism becomes slower. During these years, it is good to consider whether we are getting enough of the chemical elements needed to keep our organs working properly.

This is a time when we can think about changing our job or moving to another area. It might be good to live on the outskirts of the city to maintain a home more oriented toward wellness.

This may be a good time to develop new friends and develop a new lifestyle. Perhaps our job is taking away the time we need for exercise. A daily walk should become a necessity. Your summer vacation should be taken in a place far from work and the regular routine so that it will be a full recuperation time.

When a person has broken-down vitality, he generally has digestive problems. At this time, we have to be more careful about what we eat.

As we grow older, if we are on the pathway to disease, we end up losing the vitality of youth, and we use stimulants and aspirin to get us through the day. We have become so accustomed to taking aspirin for a headache that we don't investigate the reason for that headache, nor do we look for the causes of disease—we only attend to the symptoms.

If symptoms are ignored or suppressed, chronic conditions will set in. This is why it is important to learn about the cleansing and rebuilding needs of the body. It would be wise to consult a nutritionist to learn how to obtain the most valuable chemical balance for our particular nutritional needs. Supplements should be taken for conditions caused by stress, which can cause havoc on the body.

Western medicine is turning more toward vitamin therapy and nutritional supplementation to treat disease. The chiropractor can also be the family doctor, by integrating the use of mechanical methods and nutritional counseling in his work. The same applies for the osteopath, acupuncturist, and homeopath.

The emphasis on health during middle age is important, because at this time many people have diseases that are beginning to reach advanced stages, and they don't even realize it. Fifty percent of the people going into hospitals enter them for treatment of iatrogenic disease. This means they are being treated for the treatments they have had before. This is why I stress that suppression of symptoms by taking drugs has inevitable side effects that appear sooner or later. Cleansing methods will reverse these residual effects that drugs have left in the body and will put you on the pathway to health.

Reaping the Benefits of a Natural Lifestyle

If you have followed a natural lifestyle much of your life, you will have vigor as you get older. The benefits of a way of life that avoids symptom suppression and relies on natural foods are abundant.

If you do not stay on the natural, healthy pathway of life, your physical condition will deteriorate to the degenerative stage. In the degenerative stage, our tissue is not at a level where it can fight off or expel toxic settlements. Toxic settlements in inherently weak tissues are hampering the eliminative organs, and nature cannot perform her healing and regenerating functions. It is at this time that conditions such as arthritis, osteoporosis, emphysema, and tumors appear.

One of the most important things to consider in the chronic and degenerative stages is that all the organs will be at least 20 percent underactive by the time a person is forty-five years old, compared to age twenty-five. This is why, as we age, we get wrinkles. Older skin does not have the same pliability that younger skin has. As we grow older, we suffer with constipation, because bowel tone has become flaccid.

The degenerative stage is a dangerous one. When we were younger, we suffered with such ailments as hay fever, colds, and asthma. In the degenerative stage, we can develop cancer, heart disease, cirrhosis of the liver, and other diseases.

We all know that death cannot be avoided. But if we follow the pathway of health, we will have vitality and energy. Our old age will be enjoyable. I have always said, "A long life may not be good enough, but a good life is always long enough."

To stay on this path, we must have a daily program that revolves around our health, balanced with work, recreation, creativity, and a diet rich in whole foods that administers to every area. How many of us have creative talents that we never even touched upon because we've allowed ourselves to be "too busy"? We say we don't have enough time . . . but time is all that we have now, and we need to use that time to our advantage. Health should be at the very top of our list.

My strongest advice is to stay away from non-emergency surgery. This weakens the body. Antiseptics weaken the body.

Learn about the chemical make-up of the body. Prepare and enjoy soups and whole foods that will feed that chemical make-up and replace those lost minerals that have caused deficient conditions.

Get acquainted with salads! They can be a wealth of color and texture, and so much can be added to a salad that is delicious and health building. Food can build tissue and blood. I am not concerned with building muscles!

The world today is not set up to financially care for our aged and elderly properly. If you have children, I believe that, just as you raised and cared for them, they should reciprocate the same love and care at this time. As it is, much of the responsibility falls upon the government, and it is a great expense. We should not forget our moral responsibilities if we want a better, improved world. If we hold on to our ideals, they will keep us young, and give us courage and hope to live on.

To feel our best at any age, we need to rest and restore our body. The human body is capable of just so much within a twenty-four hour time span. Do we give ourselves enough time to repair and revitalize? Are we taking care of our nervous system so it will get us through our active days? You can compare this to winding up a clock . . . you can only wind it so much, and it will only run for so long!

The pathway to disease is one that all too many people choose to follow. But if we know how to avoid disease and want to know how good life can be, we will choose the pathway to health. It is not a difficult path to follow—and the trip is much more rewarding!

CHAPTER 7
Are We Treating Diseases or Chemical Deficiencies?

The concept of disease was developed by Western medicine to provide a convenient and useful way of cataloging human afflictions. With this system, human afflictions are identified more easily and treated more effectively.

Diseases are described in three ways. First, there are symptoms associated with each disease, including abnormal results on lab tests, x-rays, sonograms, nuclear magnetic resonance evaluations, EMI scans, and other tests. Second, there are changes in body anatomy, often verified by postmortem examination. Tissue damage always results in the course of any disease. Third, the physiology or function of some part of the body is changed. Something doesn't work right. One or more organs are unable to do their job. These are the kinds of things we associate with disease.

The American Heritage Dictionary defines disease as "an abnormal condition of an organism or part, especially as a consequence of infection, inherent weakness, or environmental stress that impairs normal physiological functioning." Notice that "infection" and "environmental stress" are considered causes of disease from *outside the body*, while "inherent weakness" is a cause of disease from *inside the body*.

The greatest tendency of Western medicine is to look for causes of disease outside the body, which are called etiological agents, or ETAs. I want to point out that when we think the cause of a disease comes from outside the body, we tend to think the cure must come from outside the body, too. So, we have a great search going on in Western medicine for more and better drugs, more refined surgical procedures and techniques, and more effective methods of chemotherapy and radiation.

In contrast, iridology and other drugless arts consider the inherent weaknesses and native constitution of the body. We see our task as taking care of the causes of symptoms to restore the body to its natural state. Correction is emphasized, not suppression. We emphasize finding and taking care of the cause of a problem.

A symptom, by itself, reveals very little about its underlying cause. There are possibly a hundred or more causes for a headache, possibly five hundred for a fever. If only the symptom is relieved or suppressed, we have done nothing to get rid of the cause.

It is well for us to ask, "What is the first domino that knocks down all the other dominoes? When we have an ache in the shoulder, what does the other 90 percent of the body tell us? Have we looked for other symptoms that may be contributing to the problem? Is there a problem with constipation or bowel regularity? Is there acidity in the body? Is calcium out of solution? What is contributing to the shoulder ache?" Many times we find that there are several causes.

EXAMINING AN AIDS PATIENT

AIDS suppresses or destroys the immune function of the body and allows every latent disease to develop. There may be ten or more diseases, other than AIDS, in an AIDS patient.

Recently, I had the opportunity to analyze the eyes of an AIDS patient. I found some interesting things with regard to his health. He had inherently weak lungs and a heavy catarrhal condition in the bronchials. His air capacity and breathing were restricted, with resulting inadequate oxygenation of the brain and body.

The iris examination revealed bowel underactivity. If the bowel is not cared for, every organ in the body will be clouded with other symptoms. His bowel transit time needed to be improved. Unless there is a fast transit time for toxic bowel materials, there is toxic reabsorption into the body. This interferes with immunity in every cell in the body, and finally backs up into the lymph system, which is the command center of the body's defense system. If the lymph system is not kept clean, we will always have disturbances and problems. This man's kidneys also were weak and not working properly.

When he was originally examined, the man was told only that he had AIDS. He was not told anything about the rest of his body. Doctors found evidence of the AIDS virus, but they didn't look further to see what the strengths and weaknesses of the body were.

One week after I told him about the lung, bowel, and kidney problems, he began to develop symptoms. Yet again, in his original examination he had not been told there was anything wrong with his lungs, bowel, or kidneys. In one week this man developed pneumonia and landed in the hospital. Pneumonia is one of the diseases that often comes with AIDS.

If there are ten diseases that accompany AIDS, why shouldn't we correct everything that we can help? If 90 percent of the body has problems other than AIDS, let's do something about it. A patient is never just sick in one part of the body. If one organ is affected, so is the rest of the body.

Let's continue with the story of this AIDS patient. One week after he got pneumonia, he developed nephritis. Where did this nephritis come from? Why didn't it show up in his original urinalysis? Did his doctors look at the inherent structure of his body? Did they have a genetic pattern to follow that would accurately show problems yet to come? Did they see what was going to break down next in the body? When I analyzed his iris, I found this pattern of genetic inheritance. With this I could see what physical problems would plague him. I also saw toxic settlements, which revealed that the kidneys would break down under the load. The kidneys could not take care of the acids, and a severe case of nephritis developed.

Why weren't these conditions discovered to begin with? Wasn't there any way to see this in the beginning? Why didn't they take care of the chemical structure of the body? Why didn't they "clean house" in the whole body? Immunity depends on the whole body working properly.

A week later the man was back in the hospital with bleeding from the bowel. Wouldn't you think that such a condition had been developing for some time? Wouldn't you suspect bowel troubles in the past? I'm wondering if we can see that this larger and very important perspective is being neglected. This is a sin of omission, a life-and-death matter. There is a lot of wisdom in considering an alternative way of handling health care by taking care of the whole body.

IRIDOLOGY REVEALS GENETIC PATTERNS

How about yourself? Is every organ in your body working at its highest point of integrity? Are your organs chemically well-balanced and toxin-free?

When the bowel, lungs and bronchials, kidneys, and skin break down, there can be many chemical shortages in the body. It takes a long time to break down these elimination channels, but if they have been on an atrocious diet, such as coffee and donuts, they will eventually break down.

The genetic patterns of people reveal a great deal. Someday, there may be a system that shows tendencies for disease in a genetic pattern. A genetic pattern, if properly interpreted, should reveal native constitution and inherent weakness. An inherent weakness in the genes shows that there is high potential for mineral deficiencies and toxic settlements. Our immune system cannot effectively protect weak organs, and an inherent weakness cannot hold chemical elements properly. Toxic material in the blood settles in the inherent weaknesses.

With iridology, we can find the inherent weaknesses and strengths in a person, and determine that person's genetic pattern. Then, we can develop a plan for that person to follow. This plan should tell us which altitude would be best to live in, the mental attitude that person should develop, the type of climate he should live in, and what type of exercise is necessary.

The key to good health is feeding our bodies with the chemical elements that inherent weaknesses have difficulty holding. We have to overfeed constantly, because the capacity of these organs for holding calcium or silica or any of the chemical elements is so poor.

A person who knows his chemical elements and knows his foods is going to treat his body using foods with the right chemical elements. Our priority is not treating AIDS, diabetes, or pneumonia. It is, first of all, recognizing where inherent weaknesses exist; second, getting rid of tissue-locked pollutions in the body; and, third, treating the chemical shortages. Those are the proper priorities in health care.

NATURAL PRINCIPLES MUST BE FOLLOWED

In countries where eating is considered an art, and where there is a cook involved in that art, degenerative diseases are most prevalent. If men and women ate more naturally, using simple, healthy foods, the majority of diseases would disappear.

As civilization has advanced, many diseases have developed, and many health arts have been developed to combat these various diseases. There is a serious compromise of health in the departure from natural principles and the taking on of unnatural habits, such as overeating, smoking, and alcohol abuse.

As it is now, the use of condiments, alcohol, coffee, tea, and bad habits such as overwork, combined with fears and other negative emotions, are endangering our health. Additionally, foul air, poor water, improper breathing, lack of exercise, loveless marriages, and many other unhealthy factors of our hypercivilization have contributed to our health problems. All these stress factors can result in the upset of our electromagnetic nerve and brain fields. The overuse of drugs, chemical sprays, artificial fertilizers, and chemical food additives contribute to the health problems that have come with our current civilization.

Unnatural lifestyles lower vitality and favor the accumulation of waste matter and poisons to such an extent that bowels, kidneys, skin, and other organs of elimination become sluggish and are unable to keep the "house" clean. Then, nature has to resort to other more radical means of purification, or we would be overcome by our own impurities. These forceable "housecleansings" of nature are colds, catarrh, phlegm, mucus, skin eruptions, diarrhea, boils, abnormal perspiration, hemorrhages, and many other forms of elimination.

SUPPRESSION IS NOT A CURE

Sulphur and coal tar medicines suppress skin eruptions, just as antihistamines, antipyretics, and pain relievers suppress cold symptoms. The doctor prescribing these medicines may congratulate himself on the speedy relief his patient experiences, but what was really accomplished? Nature has been thwarted in her work of healing and cleansing. She had to give up the fight against disease in order to combat the more potent poisons that had been taken into our body in the form of drugs. The disease and its cause are still in the system, as is the drug—or at least its residue.

When vitality has been brought back naturally, nature may make another attempt at purification, but again her well-meant efforts will be defeated. This pattern of suppression with drugs is repeated over and over again until blood and tissues become so loaded with waste material and poisons that the healing forces of the body can no longer react against them by acute responses. Chronic conditions develop, and we go still further into the incurable stage. This suppression, and the prevention of acute diseases by drugs, serums, and vaccinations, will increase instances of chronic indigestion, nervous prostration, mental disturbances, and tuberculosis. Diseases will multiply from the suppression of these problems.

It is especially unfortunate that many people acquire these diseases innocently. These drugs suppress the initial symptoms and diffuse toxic wastes throughout the system. Nature takes up the work of elimination by means of skin eruptions and ulcers in various parts of the body, but these are promptly suppressed with skin ointments. This process of suppression is continued for months or years until the body can no longer react.

THE ELIMINATION PROCESS

These conditions are verified in the iris, and the analysis of the eye reveals the presence of these poisons in the system (see my book *Case Histories in Iridology*). Many times the drug signs in the eye are accompanied by symptoms of these poisons in the system. The record in the eye is confirmed by the history of the patient. Under natural living and natural treatment, diseases that were long ago suppressed by drugs will be eliminated in healing crises. The sign in the iris will grow lighter after the healing crisis comes along. The eye will gradually be cleared of drug signs.

In natural healing, natural living, and natural treatments, as the patient improves, he becomes more vigorous until the organs of elimination act more freely. The latent poisons are stirred up from their "hiding places," so to speak. The healing crisis invigorates the organs to such an extent that an elimination process takes place. This elimination lasts several days. The elimination, brought to the surface, appears similar to symptoms of acute poisoning. The elimination process and healing crisis may be accompanied by headaches, ringing in the ears, nasal catarrh, bone pains going from joint to joint, neuritis, and a strong taste of the drug. Whenever there is a healing crisis, the signs of the disease (and the drugs used to suppress it) diminish in the iris.

This is nature's way, the key to correction of tissue, with no unwanted side effects, no long-term effects, and no time-bomb effects, as we find with drugs. Nature knows best, but sometimes she needs a helping hand.

DISEASE COMES FROM AN UNDERNOURISHED BODY

Every disease is a sign of a chemical shortage in the body. We do not feed ourselves according to chemical element needs in the body, because we are not taught to eat this way. All of these chemical elements are in our foods, but we don't know what a proper diet is. We rush through our fast food routine, living on coffee and donuts, or pickles and ice cream.

Our body tissues are saturated with food additives, chemical pollutants, and residues from all the drugs we've taken. Is it any wonder that our immunity has left us?

We have suppressed disease processes for so long that our immunity has become weaker and weaker, and we are not able to throw off the accumulated drugs and other environmental toxic material entering the body. We don't have the capacity or the potential to work properly.

A new day is going to come when we won't treat the disease. Instead, we will provide the chemical elements that a person needs. We are going to pay more attention to our chemical intake.

Doctors and people who treat chemical shortages will be considered those who give the best treatment. They will be the ones who eliminate disease, because in a well body there is no room for disease. Diseases come from an undernourished body. Bacteria and cancer develop in an undernourished body. This treatment will take time, but nature does all things in the proper time.

WHAT WE MUST KNOW IN THE FUTURE

No man should have anything to do with food preparation if he does not know the nutritional role of the chemical elements. The chemicals in every food on our shelf should be known.

We should know about soils, agriculture, animal husbandry, food processing, food storage, loss of nutrients, and what causes such losses. We should know all we can about fertilizers, pollination, and climate, and areas where the soil is lacking in certain chemical elements. We should be aware of *all* that goes into having a healthy body, and that whole, pure, and natural foods are the ideal.

People should have every bit of the organic sub-structure needed by their bodies and supplied from vegetables, fruits, nuts, seeds, and berries. Even flowers are going to be eaten in the future. What kind of an inherent background do our foods have? What pollutants are being taken in these foods today—arsenic, lead, mercury? Are any of them taken from hybrid crops? This hybrid background means a loss of the natural nutritional value that the plant had originally.

There are 270 varieties of soybeans today, and 300 varieties of avocado. Scientists are developing avocados without seeds and watermelons without seeds. The divine and original genetic patterns are being taken away from our foods, and this is destroying the immunity of plants to insect life.

We are also taking the divine genetic pattern away from human beings today by upsetting the genetic pattern with drugs. Drugs and unnatural chemicals are clouding over symptoms so that we are no longer looking at the true symptoms of the body—we are looking at accumulated drug side effects, and even genetic effects. There are drugs that have as many as sixty side effects, and we are treating these side effects as we would treat a disease. We don't treat true symptoms any more. We find our bodies are no longer normal. Patients have been drugged and polluted.

There must be a change. The dietician of the future will give the patient the chemical elements he needs so he can have a natural chemical structure restored in his or her body.

TODAY IS THE FIRST DAY OF THE AGE TO COME

It's cleanup time. Time to clean up our state of consciousness, for our knowledge and wisdom and guidance. It is time to take a turn for the better.

There is only one way to take care of this problem, and that is through cleansing the body. Fruits and vegetables are of a cleansing nature, high in sodium and potassium. These elements help neutralize the many toxic acids that develop in our bodies. There are certain kinds of foods that have an affinity for heavy metals and toxins. Chlorophyll is probably one of the greatest detoxifiers of all. The greens from the tops of vegetables have a great attraction to the metals and drug residues stored in the body. We can use foods that have been proven to have an affinity for some of these pollutants, such as Sun Chlorella. Chlorella is an edible algae with an affinity for heavy metals such as lead, cadmium, and mercury. Experiments have shown that it removes these metals from the body.

There are foods that can quicken bowel activity, and foods that can help develop a better intestinal flora, such as the friendly acidophilus bacteria. The bowel transit time can be quickened with certain foods. We have to have a certain amount of fiber. Anyone who knows nutrition will be able to tell you what foods are high in fiber and what foods serve as natural laxatives. Foods must play a central role in health in the new day to come.

FOOD—THE MEDICINE OF THE FUTURE

Nutrition is the first treatment we should consider for diseases or symptoms in the body. Whatever analysis we can get, any symptoms we encounter are going to point us to certain foods that are earmarked for that organ or disease symptom. We should know that foods have no undesirable side effects.

If our patients do not improve, we are not using the right foods to treat them. Diseases are the end result of chemically deficient organs in the body that are not functioning properly. For example, we may have different diseases produced when the liver, bronchial tubes, and stomach are not working normally together. We have another type of disease entirely when the kidneys, lungs, and small intestines are not working together properly. If the doctor didn't identify these symptoms with the conditions that caused them, the patient would never begin to heal.

We have building foods as well as cleansing foods. We have foods that regenerate, and foods that repair and rebuild. Nutritionists have developed juices and tonics to treat specific deficiencies.

We have to consider what type of analysis will be most beneficial in the use of nutrition as the medicine of the future. I don't know any better way of determining the integrity level of tissue in the body than iridology. Knowing what organs are overactive or underactive reveals what foods we need to restore chemical balance in the various organs.

Iridology has been controversial. Some have tried to compare it to a medical diagnosis, and say that it constitutes practicing medicine without a license. Many have said it is not recognized, and that is partly true. It's not recognized by the medical profession. However, iridology is recognized by hundreds of thousands of people who have benefited from it. It is recognized by many of the drugless practitioners all over the world, but it is not recognized by most of those who recommend drugs to treat disease.

Even Western medicine acknowledges the need to have tests to determine the chemicals in the blood and urine. They, too, realize that chemical imbalance is often an indication that a certain disease has developed in the body.

All the different symptoms in the body would tell us a good story. But we don't have symptoms coming from a natural body anymore. We have symptoms that are so mixed up with drugs, nostrums, and pollution chemicals that we can't get a normal symptom to express itself. I don't know if we should speak of a "normal body" anymore. There is no such thing as a normal, natural working body in this sick world today. It has been said that six out of ten people who say they feel fine these days have a chronic disease. Those who have a cancer have been twenty years in the making of that cancer. When should the doctor start looking for the problem? At the beginning, middle, or end of a disease?

Iridology enables us to see that something is wrong in the *preclinical* stage of disease. This is very important. We can tell that something is wrong in time to correct it, and with iridology, we can see when the problem is gone.

There has never before been a way of telling what foods will take care of the mineral shortages in the body. When we can find the inherent weaknesses in the body, then we know what to feed them. We know that we cannot hold full mineral values in an inherent weakness in the body. In fact, we are short of mineral elements in every inherent weakness in the body. This is what the iridologist sees, and this is what every doctor should see. This is an analysis that belongs to the nutritional field.

We are in a health revolution right this moment. Doctors are seeking answers. They are experimenting. In this age of "miracle drugs," there are more disease problems than ever. Doctors are trying to find new ways to take care of diseases that have so far resisted all treatments.

If you have a drug given to you that produces an abnormal symptom or side effect, another drug is given to you to take care of that side effect. This is a sad situation.

WE MUST LOOK BEYOND DISEASE

Iridology is not interested in disease. Iridology cannot identify particular diseases from iris signs. It is time that those who use iridology wake up to the fact that iridology is not a disease-diagnosing program. Iridology shows us where the inherent weaknesses are, what mineral development is taking place, and where shortages exist in the organs of the body. Iridology shows when a particular nutritional healing program (or other healing program) is working, and when it is not working. When tissue integrity is developed by the proper chemical elements, and regeneration has taken place with new tissue taking the place of the old, then you are on the healing path.

Those who study iridology without studying nutrition are missing the most important point. To make the changes that are necessary in tissue renewal, food is necessary. Iridology treats symptoms of inherent weakness with nutrition and *only* with nutrition.

Now, I would like to make this clear—in using iridology, we want to bring in a new body in place of the old. We are not treating symptoms. We are not trying to get rid of symptoms. When we have put new tissue in place of the old, *symptoms automatically leave of their own accord!* It may take months, but with perseverance, it will happen.

When we only take care of symptoms, we encourage a person to continue in the same disease-building consciousness that he has lived in before. He follows the same old imbalanced food program as before, stays up too late, and exercises too little. He cannot expect to put new tissue in place of the old unless he does it at the kitchen table, using the right foods in the proper proportions.

We must insist on foods that build health, not tear it down. We need more natural foods, more pure foods, more whole foods, and more raw foods. We are killing ourselves with fatty foods, fried foods, sugary foods, and junk foods.

Who will join us? People who are tired of being treated for symptom relief only, and not correction. People who are sick of being sick. People who have spent all their money on health problems, but have experienced no improvement of those problems. People who have been told, "We can't do anything for you."

WE NEED A NEW WAY OF THINKING

It is time for us to begin to think of preventive medicine. It is time that people get together and agree on the merits of a reversal system of getting well, of putting new tissue in place of the old.

Those who have taken up iridology will understand these things. Those who only take up one system in the healing art may never understand it. Those who take up the wholistic healing art should include iridology. Iridology gives them the analysis they need to work with. Iridology gives them the basis for developing new tissue from the old.

Iridology and nutrition go hand-in-hand. Without nutrition, every form of therapy, every form of treatment is incomplete. Without nutrition, tissue correction cannot take place. Do you want new tissue? What kind of tissue do you want? The same kind you have today? That's what people are going to have if they don't change their consciousness and their way of living and put in a new lifestyle in place of the old one.

It is time for us to make those changes. I appeal to those people who are seeking a godly way of life, morality in lifestyle, and a whole, pure, and natural way to live.

Those who are interested in this will join me in seeing that this philosophy is adopted in the future. I am trained in these philosophies. I know that to have this new philosophy prevail over the old disease philosophy is going to take a lot of people who stand up and say "This is the way it must be." We have lived too long with a philosophy that has resulted in more and more disease, and less and less correction. We need a change. It is time to take a higher path.

Thousands of cases have proved that my teachings will help people. Thousands of people will stand up and say this is the way they want it.

There may be millions who say you can't have it, that it isn't medically approved. There are millions who will say drugs are so much a part of our culture that we can't do without them.

There is so much opposition to the simple, beautiful way of life and health from natural nutrition that it's going to take a lot of patience and determination to make it happen.I have been preaching, teaching, and talking about these things close to fifty years. People are just beginning to become aware of these things. As far as I am concerned, we have to start with clean unpolluted nutrition. Some place, some time, that is going to happen.

It takes a truly healthy person to recognize the value of health. Often, the sick person embraces the sick way of life, defends it, and defines it as healthy. The sick person wants drugs, and wants to continue in a disease-producing lifestyle.

Are the sick going to vote against the only thing that can save their lives and restore their health? Are they sick of being sick? Let's hope so. Let's think positive, act positive, and be willing to talk to people about living a healthy way of life.

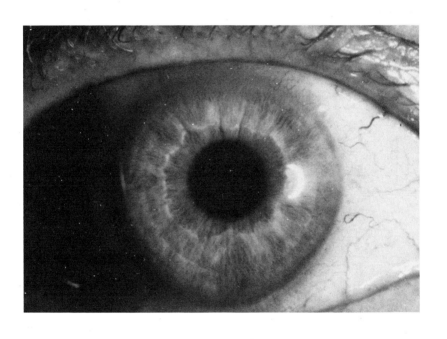

CHAPTER 8
The Miasmic Eye

In the practice of iridology, we frequently encounter patients with a dark, murky iris, indicating the long-term use of many drugs, or genetic inheritance from a parent or grandparent who used drugs heavily. We call this a "miasmic" eye. What this tells us is that drug residues and chemicals have found their way into many of the body's organs and tissues, and that a thorough tissue cleansing is needed before rejuvenation and rebuilding of tissues can take place. A miasmic eye indicates a drug-saturated, toxic body.

SOURCES OF MIASMS

Miasms can be acquired and passed on genetically from suppressant drugs and vaccinations used to treat diphtheria, malaria, tuberculosis, syphilis, cholera, plague, smallpox, typhoid, yellow fever, and other diseases. The drug profile of modern man is deplorable. Chemicals can come from so many sources.

Medicinal drugs are a multi-billion-dollar enterprise in this country, and most persons with chronic diseases have taken many powerful prescription drugs at the advice of their doctors. Our culture is drug-oriented. We take pills to wake up, pills to help us lose weight, pills for headaches, colds, and flu, pills to help us relax and pills to help us go to sleep—not to mention pills for more serious conditions. Our children are given vaccinations—even our dogs receive vaccinations.

There are people who have inherited drug residues from parents who were heavy drug users. Others have inherited genetic patterns that were either influenced by drugs or that are now influential in stimulating drug use or abuse. The minds of some people have been so altered by drugs that they don't understand what is normal or abnormal. They don't even realize that there is anything wrong with them.

Many of these people have developed into what V. G. Rocine would call a "medeic" type, a Jekyll-and-Hyde who alternates between gloom and enthusiasm. These people tend to distrust others and are prone to disregard social standards as well as the feelings of others. They may be cynical and sarcastic, ridiculing things others hold sacred, and are disease-prone.

The medeic eye looks much like a bucket of muddy water. The main problem for the iridologist is that this eye clouds the ordinary symptoms that have developed in the body, which makes it difficult to identify disease in such a person. This condition develops into iatrogenic disease.

Iatrogenic medicine, a relatively recent extension of the medical field, specializes in treating people with ailments specifically caused by the effects of drugs. It has been reported that 50 percent of hospital inpatients end up taking drugs to counteract other drugs they have taken. The drug-eyed person is the most difficult to help.

UNDESIRABLE CHEMICALS ARE EVERYWHERE

Almost every food that comes in a package, box, or can contains chemicals—artificial colors, stabilizers, thickeners, flavors, preservatives, flavor enhancers. The names may be listed on the label, but few of us have any idea what those chemicals will do once they get inside the body. Will they be broken down and excreted? Will they end up settled in the pancreas or knees? Do they have long-term effects? Personally, I prefer not to find out—not by experience, that is. Even the processing and refining of foods can alter their natural biochemical composition to render them dangerous to human health.

Chemicals are also in the local water supply. Chemicals may be added to water to destroy germ life, prevent tooth decay, settle colloidal particles, and precipitate excessive iron or other metallic compounds. Do you know what chemicals are in your drinking water? Heavy applications of agricultural chemicals and some industrial pollutants have also made their way into the ground water that people drink, cook with, and bathe in.

Industrial and auto emissions pour into the air of cities, air that must be breathed by all residents. Workers in many factories and plants breathe fumes of one kind or another for eight or nine hours a day.

Job-related exposure to chemicals is common. Photographers are exposed to powerful chemicals in their darkrooms, and the workers who make or package those chemicals are similarly exposed. Those who work in paint plants, dye factories, plastic industries, auto plants, paper mills, fertilizer plants, oil refineries—the list is almost endless—often breathe fumes and get chemicals on their skin, in their eyes and hair, and on their clothing.

Agricultural chemicals such as artificial fertilizers, weed killers, insecticides, sulphur, and other substances are sprayed or spread on the land, crops, trees, fruit, and vegetables. Farm workers are exposed, but so are those who buy these fruits and vegetables in the stores when they have not been properly washed. You can pick up an apple or cucumber in the market, and a waxy substance comes off on your hands. You can peel an orange and find that a gritty, greasy scale rubs off on your fingers.

Fish taken from the oceans are showing deposits of toxic mercury in their livers. DDT, a pesticide outlawed many years ago in this nation, is still being used by other countries, and its toxic breakdown products are found in fish, ducks, geese, and other migratory birds.

We can't escape exposure to chemicals and toxic drugs. However, some people have been exposed more than others. These people have tissues that are laden with chemicals that have not always been ingested.

Ingestion, however, is a problem. The 1960s ushered in an era of psychoactive drugs that were and are used by millions. Alcohol, nicotine, and caffeine are among the most widely-used drugs in the world. Addiction is one of the world's oldest problems, and things don't seem to be changing much. What does it take to get people to learn?

TREATMENT OF DRUG ACCUMULATIONS

Drug settlements in the body are treated the same way we would deal with any toxic condition, through the reversal process described in Hering's law of cure. We build up the strength of the tissue as much as possible through diet and exercise; we assist the elimination channels through skin brushing, herb teas, alfalfa tablets, and so on; and we may go into the seven-day tissue cleansing program to speed up the process.

Then we expectantly await the healing crisis, in which old accumulated drugs are thrown out of the body as reversal of symptoms takes place. I have been with patients during healing crises when I could smell the odor of the drug or medication taken five or ten years before, and when the patient was vividly reliving the physical symptoms and mental experiences that went along with it.

It is possible to lighten the miasmic eye and to alleviate the condition, but it can turn out to be a long-term process. It can take ten years, fifteen years, or perhaps a lifetime, to get rid of multiple drug accumulations.

THE DISCOVERIES OF NILS LILJEQUIST

In 1865, at the age of fourteen, Nils Liljequist of Stockholm, Sweden, was vaccinated and became ill. In the year following the vaccination, Liljequist developed swollen lymph glands in the neck, influenza, a racking cough, malaria, joint pains, and polyps of the nose. His doctor tried to treat the swollen lymph glands by putting iodine on the skin. The nose polyps were surgically removed, but returned year after year. He was given quinine, a drug derived from a tropical tree bark, to suppress the malaria symptoms.

During the years of these serious health problems, young Nils Liljequist noticed changes in his irides and took the trouble to keep a written
record of them. He would examine his eyes daily in a mirror, making note
of localized or general color alterations. Interestingly, Liljequist had not
heard of the discoveries of Dr. Ignatz Von Peczely in Budapest, Hungary,
and his own observations were entirely original.

Liljequist published his observations in 1871 in a paper titled, "Quinine
and Iodine Change the Color of the Iris; I formerly had blue eyes, and
they are now of a greenish color with red spots in them." Later, by studying homeopathy and using homeopathic remedies, Liljequist healed
himself.

The eye-color change from blue to green was attributed to the quinine.
The red spots (psora) in the irides were attributed to the iodine. (Psora are
localized color spots in the iris caused by drugs, while miasms change the
color of the whole iris, eventually to a dark, murky appearance.) By his
observations, the young Swedish iridologist deduced that drugs and
chemical substances could be deposited in the body tissues. (This is also
the basis of Dr. Christian Hahnemann's concept of psora as the "mother"
of disease, and led to his development of homeopathy.)

Liljequist treated many people successfully, using analysis of the iris as
a guide to selecting the appropriate homeopathic remedies. In 1893, he
published a book titled *Om Oegendiagnosen* (Diagnosis from the Eye),
thirteen years after Dr. Von Peczely published his iridology work titled
Discoveries in the Realms of Nature and the Art of Healing in Budapest.

DR. LINDLAHR AND THE HEALING CRISIS

Twenty years after Liljequist's work was published in Sweden, Dr. Henry
Lindlahr, a medical doctor in the United States, published a book titled
Nature Cure Philosophy and Practice. Lindlahr had studied iridology
with Dr. H. E. Lane (or Lahn), a native of Austria, and he was aware of
the health problems caused by psora and miasms.

Dr. Lindlahr felt that every acute stage of disease was triggered by the
body's efforts to throw off chemicals, drugs, or toxins trapped in weak
organs or tissues. Symptoms of such efforts were fever, pain, swelling,
rapid pulse, skin discharges, and catarrhal eliminations. If these were
allowed to run their course, no problem was encountered. Dr. Lindlahr
believed that suppression of these symptoms was the basic cause of more
serious problems later on in life, and he put his efforts into stimulating
elimination rather than suppressing symptoms.

"Give me a healing crisis, and I'll cure any disease," Dr. Lindlahr used
to say. He was a champion of cleansing the body through the healing
crisis, an approach first promoted by European homeopaths.

SMALLPOX VACCINE AND AIDS

Not long ago, a few nearly unnoticed newspaper articles linked the AIDS outbreak to a smallpox vaccine used by the World Health Organization in past years. The vaccine was administered to try to wipe out smallpox worldwide.

In the article, doctors who had supervised the use of the smallpox vaccine on hundreds of thousands of people in Third World countries claimed that a virus, now identified as the AIDS virus, was widespread in Africa, but was relatively harmless until the smallpox vaccine was administered. They said that this virus, once no more dangerous than the common cold, seemed to be changed into a deadly killer by its interaction with the smallpox vaccine.

This is consistent with the homeopathic theory that psora and miasmic taints alter the energy fields of body cells, causing subtle shifts in function that prepare the way for many symptoms and disease expressions. This is why it is so important to keep the body tissues clean and metabolically active.

SUPPRESSION IS DANGEROUS

Science has already discovered a drug to suppress (but not cure) genital herpes. Now, millions are being spent to find a way to stop the AIDS virus. Because of the deadly nature of this disease and the great fear it has generated, we can be reasonably certain that the greatest research effort is being made in the direction of finding a suppressive drug.

The main philosophy of treatment in Western medicine is to find the right drug to knock out the symptoms, or, alternatively, to remove a malfunctioning organ by surgery. Since surgery isn't an option in AIDS, the main research emphasis is on drugs. The great danger is that suppression of AIDS could create an even more deadly plague.

We need to turn to the philosophy of tissue correction without undesirable side effects. Physical and moral integrity are our greatest defenses against disease. We need to reevaluate our national approach to health care, increasing our emphasis on education and prevention, and recognizing that drugs are part of the problem, not the solution.

We live in a drug age, and we are creating a miasmic age for the coming years with the use of so many drugs. Unless we begin cleansing and reversing this condition, new diseases and plagues will result.

CHAPTER 9

An Alternative View of Drugs

Iridology can identify drug deposits in the body through an examination of the iris. Then, drug residues can be eliminated from the body through a cleansing process over a period of time. It may take several years for a person to become completely drug-free. As the cleansing process occurs, the iridologist can, through iris analysis, tell when the drug accumulations are gone.

The person who has drug deposits in the body will have a miasmic eye, one that is dark and cloudy. As the patient continues his cleansing-building program, he will most likely go through several healing crises over a period of time. The eyes will grow lighter, and, possibly within two years, the natural color of the eye will be restored. Many times, the scurf rim will grow smaller, showing improved elimination of the skin. The lung, bronchial, kidney, and bowel area of the iris should become lighter as elimination improves. Underactive areas in other inherent weaknesses will demonstrate that they are healing by a lighter color in the iris, and discolorations from iodine, sulphur, and quinine will begin to disappear.

DRUG POLLUTION

It is not difficult to see why so many people have the toxic drug accumulations in their bodies. I can't help but realize, as I watch television news these days, that we are in an age of drug pollution. Over the years, I've studied what drugs can do to the body. All drugs have side effects, and most of these side effects are bad news.

Side effects can be described in many different ways. They are symptoms similar to those of some diseases. These are called *undesirable* side effects, and they include diarrhea, headaches, pains, and aches. Some side effects are powerful enough to cause trouble with the heart and liver. Some drugs are sulphur-based, but the majority are derived from petrochemicals. All of these petrochemicals are considered to be potential carcinogenic agents.

We cannot expect to produce cancer the day after we have taken a petrochemical drug. It takes several years for these toxic substances to build up. Of course, those who believe in the drugs ask, "Which is worse? To have the side effects of the drugs or to continue with the health problem?"

When the side effect is death, we have to stop and consider just how far out of hand this kind of thinking has gone. For example, a recently developed sedative has been associated with forty deaths since 1986, and the FDA is just now, in 1988, being asked to look into it.

Some people experience false symptoms that are often not attributed to drugs, at least at first. The drugs cloud over the symptoms of actual diseases that the body has. Because of this, many of the analyses and diagnoses of the professionals today are false and confused, leading to inappropriate and sometimes dangerous treatments. Eventually, these people develop iatrogenic diseases. Iatrogenic diseases are so common today that 51 percent of the people who enter hospitals pick up some new disease or problem that has to be treated. In other words, they are going to be treated again for the treatment they received for their original problem.

In California, a unique "side effect" from drugs has recently been encountered by authorities. Syphilis jumped 47 percent from 1986 to 1987. Nationally, the number of cases of syphilis is up 30 percent. This is because some young women are bartering sex for rock cocaine called "crack." Crack is highly addictive, and not only will its users suffer from terribly destructive side effects down the line, but they will carry the scars of syphilis and moral compromise with them the rest of their lives.

The lymph system has become so overcrowded with toxic material that our immune systems, designed by nature to protect us from disease, are being overwhelmed. A big part of this problem is the excessive use of petrochemicals that stop the natural flow of lymph. In other words, while we are taking care of the symptoms, 90 percent of the body is being deprived of adequate lymph and adequate protection. It is about time we realize that we must take care of the whole body.

Drugs in the blood and lymph are broken down and treated like foreign substances, in many cases. The liver detoxifies them. White blood cells engulf drug particles in an attempt to protect the body from them. So, instead of enhancing our natural defenses, drugs tend to weaken them and open the door to disease.

Iridology reveals the damage that drugs are doing to our bodies, not only through psora and miasmic eyes, but through other signs. I believe that drugs and unnatural chemicals are the cause of most inflammations in the body. I believe that drugs and toxic chemicals cause the scurf rim we see in the iris, contribute to chronic bowel underactivity, and trigger glandular imbalances. Drugs compromise the integrity of our brain functions, poison the liver, interfere with digestion and assimilation, and can even cause changes in our genetic material so that the lives of the next generation become endangered. Added to the drug danger are chemical sprays, food additives, and pollutants in our air and water.

CHEMICAL DANGERS

Toxic sprays are found in the honey we buy at the store, as well as on unwashed fruits and vegetables. People have become ill and even died after using poisonous sprays on crops, lawns, and golf courses. We not only take these sprays in through the mouth and nose, but absorb them through the skin. It seems like everything in nature is being sprayed these days, and in one way or another, it comes back to us in the form of weakened bodies, disease, and death.

The major chemical companies have always had good intentions. They want to produce sprays that kill insect life, fungus, and other microorganisms that harm our food crops. They don't want to harm people. However, they don't realize that poisons strong enough to kill insects and microorganisms will also harm people. They don't realize that the excessive use of pesticides is producing genetic strains and mutant strains of insects and microorganisms that are resistant to the old chemical sprays. Experiments with the use of DDT and flies show that after several generations, a strain of flies had become immune to any amount of DDT used on them.

Perhaps, in future generations, only those human beings who have become immune to toxic chemicals will survive. This is a very sobering thought.

In our restaurants, salad bars, and supermarkets sulfite sprays are used to keep some foods fresher. A number of people have become ill, and several have died from these sprays. Flavor-enhancing chemicals such as monosodium glutamate are often used in restaurants. I have to admit these fresh-looking foods look very tempting, but what goes along with them is very dangerous.

Our soil has become so drenched and polluted with chemicals that natural seeds cannot even grow in some soils today. We are using unnatural hybrid seeds to produce food crops that look wonderful and have a longer "shelf live" at the store, but are lacking in nutrients.

Nearly 30 percent of the water systems in the United States are contaminated by agricultural chemicals, according to government tests. Radon, an odorless, radioactive gas that percolates into buildings from underground rocks, is estimated to be responsible for 13,000 lung cancer deaths each year.

CAFFEINE, NICOTINE, AND ALCOHOL

Caffeine, nicotine, and alcohol are the most widely abused drugs in the world. I wonder if we realize that caffeine can destroy the calcium-holding power in the body? Pregnant women who drink coffee risk a calcium deficiency in the child they are carrying. Alcohol is now definitely known to cause brain damage in unborn children, and destroys the brain cells of those who use it. Nicotine causes dramatic physiological changes in the body. This is described in detail in the Surgeon General's Report on Smoking, published many years ago. The worst side effect of nicotine is lung cancer. We must realize that not only are excessive use of nicotine and alcohol linked to heart disease and cancer, but they weaken the liver, and are capable of combining with other chemical pollutants and drug residues in the body to form deadly poisons and carcinogens. If caffeine, nicotine, and alcohol were immediately dropped by everyone in the United States, I'd expect at least a 20 percent improvement in health.

HEAVY METAL PROBLEMS

An examination of the iris doesn't reveal toxic concentrations of heavy metals in the organs, but the effects of these concentrations are seen in the subacute, chronic, and degenerative lesions. An excess of mercury in our bodies can come from the fillings in our teeth. Mercury was used to cure syphilis in the past, and was passed on from generation to generation as a psoric taint. The dangers of mercury were confirmed in England years ago. Hat makers in this country once used mercury in their hats to give the brim a nice form. But the men who made these hats had to breathe the fumes, and in a matter of a few years brain damage caused them to go crazy, and they were taken off to mental institutions. That is why they were called the "mad hatters!"

DRUGS, CHEMICALS, AND YOUR CHILDREN

It is not just happenstance that Dr. Goldfine, of the Kaiser Clinic in Oakland, California, found that salicylates in drugs and foods were causing hyperactivity in children. This is just another symptom, another side effect. Why don't we stop and listen and see just what is going on?

Sulphur drugs have been used over so many decades that the drug effects are passed from generation to generation. We are living in drugged bodies. Purity cannot come from impurity. Pure children cannot come from impure parents. Drugs have gone into the fourth generation, and if we are not careful, we will not have any generations in the future. Man is destroying himself. Today's generation must make an about-face, or there will come a point when there is no place to turn around.

Take the example of thalidomide. Mothers who took this drug during their pregnancy bore children who had no arms or legs. The company that produced the drug settled for millions of dollars, and stopped producing the drug. However, many companies are still making drugs that produce birth defects.

WHO IS RESPONSIBLE FOR YOUR HEALTH?

I haven't seen a strong, naturally healthy person in a long, long time. Every person who comes in to see me has at least ten things wrong with him. Most of my patients have spent years going to doctors who gave them drugs, and after short periods of symptom relief, they had recurrences of their problems, some worse than before.

Of course, people who complain of aches and pains are just as much at fault as doctors who advocate drugs to get rid of the symptoms. People demand drugs because they don't want to go to work when they have a headache. School officials don't want a coughing, sneezing child in the classroom. This is why we are bombarded with advertising that "pushes" drugs and advocates the suppression of symptoms.

THE "RELIEF SOCIETY"

We are living in a "relief society." This "relief society" gets rid of your pain just to keep you on the job, giving you stimulation to keep you going and a sedative at night to help you sleep. These drugs are made from petrochemicals that are cancer forming, and in the next twenty years, you may find yourself in a chronic or degenerative disease. The "relief society" of today is really the motivating force behind the chronic diseases and degenerative problems that man has developed.

Once, drugs were advertised that stopped catarrhal drainage for six hours. Now there are drugs that stop it for twelve. There are drugs to suppress allergy symptoms. Our country has gone wild over treating allergies. They say allergies are the beginning of heart problems, lung disturbances, or rheumatism. Allergies can be indicated by coughs, hives, sniffles, postnasal drip, stuffed-up sinuses, and sneezing.

What most people don't realize is that allergies can be triggered by the drugs we have taken. Environmental chemicals also cause allergies. The chemical spray used on alfalfa is eaten by the cow, goes into the milk, onto the table, and ends up in us. These sprays have produced a lot of allergic reactions in people.

The greatest health problem of our time is the suppression of acute symptoms, because suppression increases both the chance of getting a disease and the severity of a disease. In my view, suppression is the basic cause of 90 percent of the chronic diseases of our time. To use drugs only for relief of symptoms is a form of self-poisoning, a slow and shameful suicide.

I am not opposed to drugs used to relieve extreme pain or save lives. This is a legitimate and justifiable application. However, I oppose the use of drugs in any condition where an alternative treatment is available.

We are certainly in a dilemma. With each drug discovered, we are killing ourselves off a little more. The problem is that each new drug given to people combines in the body with old residues from drugs taken in the past, or interacts wih psoric taints inherited from previous generations. This brings about unpredictable chemical combinations in the body that can have unpredictable side effects, long-term effects, and time-bomb effects. The result may be cancer or kidney failure. It may be insanity, Alzheimer's disease, or glandular dysfunction.

It isn't one cup of coffee that causes death, or one piece of chocolate that kills us, or one glass of orange juice that helps us. Doing the wrong thing for a long period of time, however, eventually brings disease. Then we are going to have to do the right thing for years to restore our health.

We need to turn this problem around and start thinking in terms of cleaning up our act, physically and mentally. A drug that shows no side effects in a person at the age of twenty-five may cause horrible side effects when he takes it again at the age of thirty-five, because body chemistry changes. We need to start thinking of eliminating drugs from our lives completely, or at least, as much as possible.

CHAPTER 10
Modern Plagues:
Herpes II and AIDS

Suppressive drugs have been used to treat the vast epidemics of syphilis, gonorrhea, and other sexually-transmitted diseases over the past forty years. This has resulted in a new and more powerful danger to those who may have had several treatments with these drugs, because the venereal taint that has made them vulnerable to sexually-transmitted diseases has been driven deeper and become more highly concentrated.

Not many years ago, we saw the initial consequences of this suppression—a new (or relatively new) sexually-transmitted disease. This disease was really not new, but was commonly known as herpes, a viral disease that doctors were accustomed to treating around the mouth. Only this time, the blisters and sores characteristic of this viral disease were being found around the genitalia and the anus. The blisters and underlying condition went through periodic cycles of pain and itching that were almost unbearable. It was an extremely embarrassing and painful disease. Continued sexual relations would pass the disease to each sex partner.

Because it showed up in a different location from the original herpes (around the mouth), the early disease was called Herpes I and the newest version was called Herpes II. Unfortunately, there was no cure. After a year or two of frantic research, however, researchers came up with a symptom-suppressive drug that stopped the worst of the symptoms.

Of course, the danger was evident. The new sexually-transmitted disease called Herpes II was brought into existence by suppression of other sexually-transmitted diseases. Now it, too, was being suppressed by another drug. I can't tell you how devastating this is to the immune system and the natural defenses of the body.

Possibly the most important lesson to be learned from these attempts to wipe out sexually-transmitted diseases, including the latest epidemics—Herpes II and AIDS—is the failure to deal with the causes: sexual promiscuity, irresponsible lifestyle, immorality, unhealthy marriages, and out-of-control sexually compulsive behaviors. Experts are writing articles and books these days about "sexual addiction," putting it in the same category as alcoholism or drug addiction. I agree with this idea. Any out-of-control behavior actually signals the presence of mental and physical deficiencies that need treatment.

After several years of Herpes II, AIDS (Acquired Immune Deficiency Syndrome) emerged. This is a killer disease that is transmitted by body fluids through sexual intercourse or contaminated hypodermic needles (and other less common practices). AIDS came out soon after treatments began on the Herpes II syndrome.

AIDS is more deadly than Herpes II. It attacks and destroys the immune system, so that any other disease—such as pneumonia, Herpes II, or cancer—multiplies out of control in the patient, and leads to death. Another unusual aspect of AIDS is that it can be carried in a contagious state for years without any symptoms in the carrier, so that dozens or hundreds of sexual partners can become infected.

So far, no one who has shown active symptoms of AIDS has survived more than a few years. It is not so far-fetched to say that we have two modern plagues on our hands—Herpes II and AIDS. Even though Herpes II can be controlled, it is not being eliminated. Once you have it, you keep it.

There is no cure for AIDS, and the number of cases is expected to increase 50 percent this year over last year. This disease is worldwide. Scientists may not find a satisfactory suppressive drug or therapy for AIDS, because the destruction of the immune system may not be reversible. Death comes relatively soon after symptoms appear. AIDS has become an extreme epidemic. Great numbers of people are involved.

WHAT COULD HAVE CAUSED AIDS?

I understand that AIDS is passed along from person to person by a deadly virus, but where was this virus twenty years ago? Where was AIDS thirty years ago? Why did it come in our time?

I believe AIDS comes from the use of drugs in the suppression of many of our diseases, all the way back to childhood diseases, and it is reinforced or confirmed or invited by continuing on in the same lifestyle that brought those diseases to us in the first place. No disease can be said to be cured unless the damaged or infected tissue is replaced by healthy new tissue, and drugs don't do that. I don't believe you can find a doctor in this world who will tell you that drugs can build new tissue. They can only suppress symptoms, and suppression is not a cure, even though the symptoms may be gone.

Suppression of disease by drugs or other means appears to weaken or break down the immune system. The lymphatic system depends on the four elimination channels to be toxin-free and clean. The lymph fluid visits every organ in the body. There is three times as much lymph fluid in the body as there is blood, and it reaches the most intricate parts of the body to bring nutrients to the tissues and to carry away toxic waste. It is one of the two most important fluids that exist within the body. It carries nourishment in and wastes out, and when it is stopped by congestion, our tissues are flooded with acid wastes. This condition makes us susceptible to disease.

The environment has become so laden with toxic substances that it contributes to the breakdown of the immune system. We take in carbon monoxide, lead, pesticide residues, food additives, cleaning solvents, paint fumes, and who knows what else! Whenever people have the slightest cold, the slightest discharge, they use cold remedies and cough syrups that suppress symptoms. Even skin lotions, cosmetics, and hair dyes add to the chemical burden of the body. These all accumulate and produce side effects, as all drugs do in the body.

Pollution in the air and water, degerminated, refined foods, lack of exercise, high-stress jobs, and fast-lane lives are leading us to a disease problem. Our bodies are starving for essential minerals. We no longer use whole, pure, and natural foods. I believe that a plague comes easily to starving people. AIDS is exploding in Africa, and it's coming to the rest of the world as well.

The pathway to disease involves progressive stages of tissue inactivity, from acute to subacute to chronic to degenerative. Once emphysema and cancer were classified as degenerative stages of disease, but they are not as degenerate as AIDS. With AIDS, there is, at the present time, no hope for a cure.

WHAT CAN WE LEARN FROM HERPES AND AIDS?

The integrity of brain/mind function is closely related to the history of contamination of the body. Drugs, pollution, use of alcohol and tobacco, food additives, and other unnatural chemicals alter tissue structure and function.

The Center of Broca and other areas of the brain related to speech and language structure are essential to our concepts of past, present, and future. When brain function is altered or depleted beyond a certain point, a person begins to lose that higher sense of destiny which marks the best side of the human race. He begins to revert to the animal nature. The lower level of consciousness dominates, and life becomes a constant hunt for sex and food.

When sex, instead of the good of others, becomes the highest goal in life, this is an indication of a disease state at the mental and moral levels. AIDS and Herpes II are only outward manifestations of an existing internal morality. The integrity of mind and morals were deficient and toxic-laden *before* the body was deficient and toxic laden. As we know, the body follows the mind—until the mind becomes unable to lead. After that, the mind follows the body, to the downfall of both.

I understand that innocent men, women, and children have contracted AIDS and Herpes II through no fault of their own. However, it appears from the evidence at hand that they make up a very small percentage of the total number afflicted.

From AIDS and Herpes II we should understand the need for wholistic integrity—integrity of body, mind, and spirit. It is time to reverse the trend that is destroying the best things in man. The higher ideals and goals that lead to peace on earth and goodwill to all men should be the trend to follow.

We must have a massive cleaning-up program throughout the world. We need to straighten up our act and come back to the natural and moral principles that have made nations and cultures strong, healthy, orderly, creative, peaceable, and productive in the past.

Who is going to teach the world what it desperately needs to hear? Will you be one of those who points the way to a higher path when people ask you what to do? If you won't do it, who will?

CHAPTER 11

Men and Women:
Their Different Health Needs

Not long ago, a study published by a major medical institute claimed that over 9 million unnecessary surgeries were performed on women during the preceding year. A significant percentage of those were hysterectomies. Another study reported that nearly 80 percent of the men over age sixty have had prostate operations. Heart disease is far more prevalent in men than women (women seem to be protected by female hormones until menopause), but women have more bowel problems than men by a ratio of two to one. Among cancer fatality statistics, the leading cause of death among men is lung cancer (33 percent) while the leading cause among women is breast cancer (11 percent). Women account for 70 percent of all cases of rheumatoid arthritis. More men become alcoholics and develop cirrhosis of the liver than women. Osteoporosis is epidemic among older women.

We find in the preceding statistics and percentages that significant differences exist in the extent and types of diseases that afflict men and women. In this chapter, we will explore some of the reasons for these differences and what can be done about them. Over the past fifty years, I have had the opportunity to listen to the health complaints of thousands of men and women, and these, together with what iridology has revealed about tissue conditions in their bodies, have led me to certain conclusions.

For many years, I traveled to different parts of the world, searching for the secrets of health and longevity. I found a considerable number of people in the age range of 100 to 160 years, and most of them were men. In the United States, however, women live an average of eight years longer than men, and this gave me something to think about. There are differences between our culture in the United States and other cultures that can teach us some useful lessons regarding health.

CULTURAL HEALTH DIFFERENCES

Three of the most important health-related differences between our culture and others I studied in which a significant number of people lived to a ripe old age, free of disease, are these: first, the people ate more complex carbohydrates—fruits, vegetables, whole grains, nuts, and seeds—and less meat than the people of this country. Second, they ate less than the average American. Third, they were more physically active. This third difference is the key to why men tended to live longer than women in the various cultural groups I visited (such as the Hunzas, the people of the Caucasus mountains in the Soviet Union, and the Turks).

In many of these places, both men and women worked actively out-of-doors for much of their lives. But women spent more time indoors, raising children and taking care of household chores. At some point around the age of sixty, the women would withdraw into their homes to focus primarily on household chores, while the men still worked in the fields, bending, stooping, lifting, and walking a great deal in and around the hills and mountainsides. I believe this extra activity on the part of the men kept their hearts strong, their blood and lymph flowing well, and their minds clear and alert. This is extremely important in maintaining good health.

Much of American life for both sexes is sedentary. We sit to do our work, drive our cars, watch television, and eat our meals. Do American women who are responsible for the upkeep of a home get more exercise than their husbands who hold desk jobs? An interesting question. However, the majority of Americans of both sexes are overweight, and obesity is a major health hazard in the United States.

In the United States, women tend to see their doctors sooner and more often than men when they have health complaints. They follow the doctor's instructions more carefully and faithfully and seem to be more conscious of what they eat. American men do not take care of themselves as well as they should. They allow physical problems to go on for too long before seeking professional help. Because of this attitude, men often develop more serious, chronic problems than women, and this should be remembered when working with men.

We find that the vigorous, energetic male who "feels good" is most neglectful of his health. He usually treats his body more harshly than women treat theirs. He may overwork himself, drink too much, compete too strenuously with other men, overexert himself in sports and exercise when he is out of shape, eat too much, and stay up too late. Men are prone to ignore cuts, fevers, infections, sore throats, colds, and dental problems unless they are in pain. Few men get sufficient, regular exercise or appropriate relaxation. The average over-forty American male is flabby, overweight, underexercised, and eats too much fatty, salted meat. Many have high blood pressure and hardening of the arteries.

Women tend to talk about what worries them much more than men, and to express their emotions more freely. Men internalize their feelings, hold their anger, and cover up their worries. (Men also get ulcers more often than women, primarily for this reason.)

WHAT IRIDOLOGY SHOWS ABOUT MEN AND WOMEN

Iridology, the science of reading tissue conditions in the iris of the eye, reveals what is essentially the health history of the individual. It shows the inherent strengths and weaknesses of the various organs and systems, and whether inflammation is present in any part of the body. We can see signs of anemia, lymphatic congestion, nerve stress, and drug deposits in the eye. From the degree of darkness in portions of the iris, we can interpret the degree of tissue degeneration in parts of the body and tell whether the condition is long-standing or relatively recent.

When we see signs of lymphatic congestion in the iris, we consider several factors. Are the food habits of the person creating catarrh in the body? Is the person getting enough exercise to clear out catarrh and move the lymph along? Is the bowel throwing too much toxic material into the bloodstream for the body's immune system to handle? Are any of the eliminative channels underactive, causing catarrh to gather because it can't be eliminated fast enough?

Because the breasts are primarily made up of lymph tissue, lymph blockage can cause problems ranging from minor lumps to more serious degenerative conditions. Estrogen from oral contraceptives and high cholesterol foods is thought by doctors to increase the chances of breast cancer, which makes it worthwhile for women to examine their breasts regularly and inform their doctors of any abnormal findings. (See Figure 11.1.) The breasts should be examined a week after the period each month, and examinations should be continued after menopause.

We cannot identify disease from the signs in the iris, but we can distinguish the conditions that contribute to disease. For example, when we discover a dark gray or black lesion in the liver area of the iris, there is no way of telling whether it is hepatitis, cirrhosis, or another disease. What we know is that a serious level of inflammation and degeneration is taking place in the liver, and that is sufficient to indicate what must be done, in conjunction with the other problems revealed in the iris and the care they require. We always take care of the whole body, never only the symptoms of one organ.

When we observe inherent weakness showing some stage of tissue inflammation—acute, subacute, chronic, or degenerative—we know immediately there is a chemical deficiency in that organ or tissue. If we see inflammation in the thyroid area, we know the body needs iodine. If we see inflammation in the gastrointestinal area, we know the body needs sodium. This is all explained in more detail in the chapter on iridology and nutrition. Our point is simply that, from what we see in the iris, we know what parts of the body are suffering chemical deficiencies, how serious the deficiencies are, and the chronological or sequential order in which the deficiencies have developed.

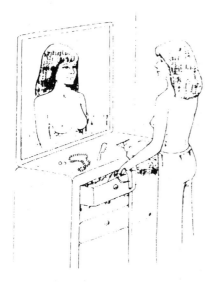

Examine your breasts regularly to check for any lump, hard knot, or thickening. Learn to recognize the normal contours of your breasts, and ask your doctor to confirm your findings during your next visit. If you feel any new lumps or any lumps that have enlarged, promptly report this to your doctor.

1. Look at your breasts in the mirror, first with your arms at your sides, and then with your arms above your head. Look for changes in the appearance of the breasts or nipples, such as a swelling or dimpling of the skin.

2. Place your arms at your side. Keeping your fingers flat, gently palpate one breast with the opposite hand by moving the hand in a circular motion over the entire breast area. You may wish to do this during a bath or shower, as your fingers will then glide easily over the wet skin. Repeat the procedure on the second breast. Then, with arms raised, repeat the procedure again. While your arms are raised, carefully palpate the nipple area and the tissue lying under it.

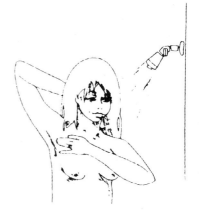

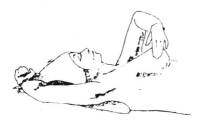

3. Lie flat on your back with a pillow or folded towel placed under your shoulder on the first side that is to be examined. Using the same circular motion described earlier, check the texture of your breast. Move the towel or pillow to the other shoulder, and repeat the procedure.

Figure 11.1   Breast Self-Examination

Depleted tissue is unable to eliminate toxic waste, whether this consists of metabolic waste, catarrh, toxins from the blood, or drug settlements. As a result, cellular activity becomes devitalized, nerve impulses are inhibited, and conditions become ripe for serious illness and chronic disease to set in. This is how men and women develop the host of maladies to which a seemingly endless list of disease names are attached.

We do not find well-defined differences between the eyes of men and women in iridology. We may see a greater tendency to anemia of the extremities in women, a weaker tissue structure in the muscles, and perhaps more thyroid conditions. We may find a greater degree of darkness in the bowel area, more hardening of the arteries, and coarser structure in the joints and ligaments of men. Despite known differences in the frequency, type, and severity of certain diseases between women and men, it appears very much that the same basic causes give rise to somewhat different disease manifestations because of differences in hormones, sex organs, reproductive functions, social roles, and lifestyles. For example, women are protected from arteriosclerosis and other manifestations of cardiovascular disease by the female hormone estrogen, even though they share the same fatty diet and similar lifestyle habits as men.

It is not possible to determine the sex of an individual from the iris. Notice in the chart arrangement how male and female organs are represented in the same locations. (See Figure 3.1 on page oo.)

FOUR MAJOR CAUSES OF DISEASE

From the iridologist's point of view, there are four major causes for men's and women's diseases: lack of exercise, faulty nutrition, gravitational effects, and nerve depletion.

Insufficient Exercise and the Lymph System

Exercise is necessary for the lymph system to flow. Chronic lymph congestion can open the door to chronic disease. There are about forty pints of lymph fluid in the body, as compared to an average of fifteen pints of blood. Lymph reaches tissues and performs functions that the blood does not, and keeping the lymph fluid clean and in motion is one of the keys to good health. Figure 11.2 shows the places in the body that can be affected when lymph fluid contains toxic accumulations.

Poor diet and excess use of refined carbohydrates are responsible for the overacidity the iridologist sees in the majority of women's eyes. Americans also use far too much of the milk and wheat products in their diet—54 percent of their entire food intake. These are acid- and catarrh-forming foods, contributing to respiratory problems and a general excess of catarrh in the body that can lead to cysts, lymph node engorgement,

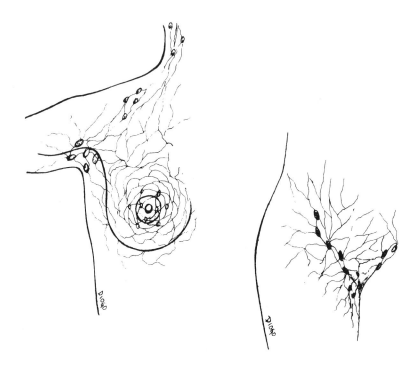

Figure 11.2   The Lymph System

Lymph tissue concentrations in the axilla (armpit) and breast (*left*), and groin (*right*). When lymph fluid becomes congested with toxic accumulations and is not eliminating properly, enlargements and cystic conditions can develop in these organs.

and inflammations. Catarrh irritates the tissue it touches; that is why we eliminate rather than suppress it.

Poor Food Habits

Poor food habits and lack of exercise also contribute to constipation, in which the contents of the bowel are held too long before elimination. This allows transference of toxic materials through the bowel wall and into the bloodstream and lymph system, contributing to toxic conditions elsewhere in the body, but most particularly the pelvic region. Constipation due to faulty nutrition and lack of exercise, together with prolapsus of the transverse colon, may create a potentially dangerous situation. When ovarian, uterine, or prostatic cysts and tumors develop, drainage is so impaired that if the condition is not taken care of, degenerate tissue may develop. Constipation also places a much greater burden on other elimination organs, such as the kidneys.

Gravity

Gravity is a major cause of colon prolapsus, which generates pelvic problems in men and women. As an ever-present force that pulls on the body constantly, we tend to get used to it and take it for granted. Yet, we must realize that the venous blood in the legs must work against gravity to get back to the heart. Gravity plays a role in all circulatory and anemia problems, and the cilia of the lungs must also work against it to eliminate catarrh and foreign matter.

Nerve Depletion

Depletion is a common ailment among those who have high-stress-producing jobs, marriages, and relationships, and who don't know how to take care of the nerves through proper nutrition and relaxation. The nerves need phosphorus, calcium, magnesium, and silicon. We must get an adequate supply of the nerve fats, cholesterol, and lecithin. Usually we get all the cholesterol we need (sometimes far too much), so it is lecithin we must pay attention to. We often destroy lecithin by overcooking, and our primary sources are nuts, seeds, whole grains, and egg yolk. Raw egg yolk in black cherry juice is a wonderful nerve tonic. Without the proper nerve supply to the organs, glands, and tissues, the central nervous system control cannot help stimulate healing, chemical balancing, and so forth.

In all developing problems in the body, iridology offers the only means of finding inflammation and chemical imbalance before symptoms appear. Early treatment can prevent chronic conditions and disease.

SEXUALLY TRANSMITTED DISEASES

Sexually transmitted diseases rose to epidemic proportions in both men and women in the United States in the 1970s because of a shift in moral values among young people. There is much more to sex than the physical side of it, and the high risk of infection should give young people something to think about. Spiritual and mental principles and laws cannot be forgotten in our relationships with other human beings.

The most surprising aspect of the venereal disease epidemic is the outbreak of Herpes II, a virus transmitted by sexual contact, which erupts in often painful blisters and ulcers around the sex organs; and AIDS, a fatal disease that destroys the immune system.

By 1982, over 5 million Americans had herpes. Once contracted, the outbreak of symptoms may occur any time, lasting usually from five to seven days. Doctors have found that L-lysine relieves acute symptoms and prevents recurrent outbreaks when foods high in argenine are avoided. Argenine makes the herpes virus multiply rapidly, and is found in foods such as nuts, chocolate, and peanut butter.

AIDS is primarily transmitted by sexual contact, especially anal sex, and by blood infection (most frequently by addicts who share needles). Presently, it is epidemic in gay men. Babies born to mothers who have AIDS also have AIDS. The most dangerous thing about the AIDS virus is that no symptoms appear for many years, but the disease can still be passed along to others without anyone realizing what is happening.

COLON PROLAPSUS AND PELVIC PROBLEMS

Of special interest are the profoundly different ways in which prolapsus of the transverse colon affects men and women. The transverse colon is represented by the area from eleven to one o'clock in both eyes, just inside the autonomic nerve wreath. A dip toward the pupil in this part of the iris indicates prolapsus, and we can easily observe its effects on the pelvic region and its glands and organs through iridology analysis.

Prolapsus may interfere with fluid transmission from the bowel to the bloodstream and lymphatic system. It always interferes to some degree with circulation and nerve supply to the pelvic organs, reducing the nutrient supply, waste elimination, and normal nerve response. A dropped transverse colon causes pressure on the ovaries, ovarian tubes, uterus, bladder, sigmoid colon, and rectum in women, which may produce menstrual problems, tipped uterus, sterility, ovarian cysts, infections of the uterus and bladder, and hemorrhoids. Because wastes cannot be carried away normally from this region by compressed blood and lymph vessels, toxic accumulations complicate the pressure symptoms, contributing to infections and chronic conditions. Additionally, problems due to prolapsus will affect the brain area, reducing the efficiency of brain functions.

In men, the prolapsus presses against the prostate gland, bladder, sigmoid colon, and rectum. Prostate infections, enlargement, and tumors may result, as well as hemorrhoids, bladder infections, and impeded blood and lymph supply to the testes.

Not all prolapsus symptoms are as dramatic as those previously described. Prolapsus pressure may, for some time, generate only a mild discomfort in the pelvic area or groin, with possible leg pains. More serious problems develop, however, as time goes by and the condition is not taken care of.

Prolapsus is caused, I believe, by calcium deficiency together with fatigue problems. It is a gravity-related condition, and the tissue that holds the transverse colon in place can't do its job without the right nutrients and rest. Calcium strengthens tissue. What we do to relieve prolapsus symptoms are slant board exercises, which reverse the effects of gravity.

Among women, pressure on the ovaries may interfere with estrogen production, throwing off the menstrual cycle and altering normal body chemistry. Among men, pressure on the prostate may interfere with the production of the alkaline fluid that helps protect the spermatazoa. Sterility in either men or women can result from prolapsus. The diminished blood supply to the pelvic area may also affect testosterone production in men, interfering with normal body chemistry.

WOMEN'S REPRODUCTIVE PROBLEMS

At the outset of this chapter, we remarked about the many reportedly unnecessary female operations performed each year, a high percentage of them hysterectomies. Doctors tend to recommend hysterectomies when they have exhausted their limited arsenal of pills for female problems, and when the symptoms and complaints persist. One of the least visible sources of female problems is prolapsus of the transverse colon, but others include diverticula and constipation (both of which may be accompanied by prolapsus). These are correctable or subject to improvement, in any case. I am not suggesting that all female operations are unnecessary, but it is clear that many doctors need to develop a greater awareness of various treatments they can recommend before resorting to surgery.

Tissue cleansing and bowel management, together with dietary measures, are basic approaches that often help in cases of female problems. Slant board exercises will greatly alleviate prolapsus problems. A University of California study has shown that constipated women (those who had two or fewer bowel movements per week) were much more likely to have abnormal cells associated with cancer in their breasts than those who had daily bowel movements, and other studies have indicated that twice as many women as men have irritable bowel syndrome (IBS). Chronic constipation often results from a diet high in protein, fat, refined flour products, and sugar, and low in whole grains, fruits, and vegetables. It also helps to take two teaspoons of wheat bran and four alfalfa tablets after each meal to increase bowel bulk, speed up movement of waste, and feed beneficial bowel flora. It is my impression that women who report problems with constipation also report more frequent and severe female problems, including menstrual difficulties and infections. One of the first considerations in problems with the female organs or processes is to take care of constipation.

Premenstrual difficulties—cramps, bloating, skin eruptions, depression, anger, temper and nerve problems, headaches—may be caused by a lack of progesterone, as suggested by Dr. Katharina Dalton, or they may be related to bowel problems, as previously described. Supplemental calcium and vitamin D, together with an herbal diuretic tea and vitamin B-6 for the bloating, have worked well for many women.

Prolonged menstruation, with or without cramps, can usually be corrected by suitable doses of vitamin E. When the flow is excessive, includes dark clots, and is followed by spotting, black cohosh and licorice are often very helpful, best in the form of tea but also effective in capsules. Menstrual problems linked with a subnormal temperature may indicate thyroid hypoactivity. When dulse tablets are taken and the thyroid improves, the menstrual problems, in such cases, often disappear. Keep in mind that menstrual blood is forty times higher in calcium than normal blood. The calcium and iron lost during menstruation must be replaced; calcium deficiency is one cause of cramps.

Women with a history of miscarriages and stillbirths have often responded well to supplements of dulse and vitamin E. Dr. John A. Myers has claimed that iodine deficiency is frequently associated with miscarriage or stillbirths.

Endometriosis is caused when a portion of the endometrium, which is normally sloughed off during menstruation, finds its way back up the fallopian tubes. The tissue remains "alive," growing in response to rising estrogen levels each month. It can cause ovarian cysts, urinary problems, bowel obstructions, infertility, and other problems. Because the endometrial tissue grows larger with time, it may be mistaken for cancer and treated as such by doctors. Endometriosis is difficult to detect because it mimics so many of the symptoms of female problems with other causes. However, its main early symptoms are abdominal pain, tenderness before and after periods, abnormally long periods, painful bowel movements, and abnormal pain during the digestive process. It is now thought that endometriosis may be relatively common.

One of the major health-impacting events women encounter is pregnancy. This is often a time when the body chemistry is tested to its fullest, since the growing fetus draws all its nutrients from the mother's body. This is when many women become depleted of calcium, iron, and other biochemical nutrients, and their health suffers terribly in subsequent years. It doesn't have to happen. By preparing for pregnancy using a good food regimen to cleanse and build a healthy body, a woman can assure herself and her child of adequate reserves of chemical elements throughout the term of pregnancy and afterward. Iodine, manganese, calcium, copper, and zinc are very important elements in reproduction and healthy pregnancies, and are among the most common deficiencies.

Menopause, the time-of-life change in women, can be another troublesome time. For some women, the process takes place very quickly, and without complications; for others, it drags on for years with many difficult and problematic symptoms. Estrogen treatments may sometimes be justified, but their link with degenerative disease is so well established that the reasons for using the estrogen must be extreme. According to Dr. Roy Hertz, MD, of the National Institute of Health, "We know that estrogens, when given in large doses over a prolonged period, will induce tumors of breast, cervix, endometrium, pituitary, testicles, kidney, and bone marrow in mice, rats, rabbits, hamsters, and dogs." Dr. Hertz believes the results of the animal studies also apply to man.

Birth control pills, we should realize, are also made of steroid hormones. Studies have shown that these hormones are linked to cancer.

There are many other factors that contribute to the physical problems of women. In particular, high-heeled shoes cause lumboscaral spine trouble, tampons cause toxic absorptions, contraceptives reduce mental efficiency, nylon clothing holds high bacterial counts, cosmetics and hair dyes cause irritation and chemical absorption, and tight bras and girdles cut off circulation and respiration.

Both men and women err in not taking time off to do the things they love to do, or to relax and recover from family duties. Many in both sexes lack the spiritual guidance and teaching to lead inspired, uplifted lives.

ESPECIALLY FOR MEN

Among men, it is possible to note a correlation between an underactive, toxic bowel and arteriosclerosis, a common cardiovascular disease. Poor food habits contribute simultaneously to the toxic bowel condition, to constipation, and to the contents of the bloodstream that create arterial and other lesions in hardening of the arteries. Excessive salt use, smoking, and heavy alcohol use also contribute to this disease.

As toxic, acidic conditions begin to develop in the body, changes may be noted in the sex life. Right or wrong, many men measure their lives in relation to their sexual activities, including problems and dysfunctions. The beginnings of sexual dysfunction can be detected most effectively with iridology. Toxic and acidic conditions, nerve stress, and a toxic bowel can be detected before chemical changes seriously disrupt the hormonal levels and balance.

High blood pressure arises when we have not found a right way of living. Blood pressure mounts when job and home stresses are not constructively handled and when men indulge excessively in drinking, smoking, salt intake, and fatty meats, especially pork and beef. I recommend cutting down on red meat, which tends to putrefy easily in the bowel.

I encounter many men and women whose adult health problems are an outgrowth of childhood conditions that were never properly taken care of. Perhaps the tonsils were taken out, but the condition that caused the tonsillitis was never dealt with. Then came appendicitis, or maybe cavities in the teeth, skin eruptions, or acne. The lymph system is congested and toxic, yet we've never done anything about it. As midlife approaches, we are faced with the need to deal with these long-neglected problems, or pay the price of ongoing chronic or degenerative disease.

Often, men are the engineers and mechanics in our society. They would never think of putting the wrong fuel in a car or plane. They would strenuously object to inadequate maintenance or poor repair. Why, then, do they neglect the most important piece of equipment in anyone's life—the human body? Why do they think the most fabulous machine of all can take excessive punishment and neglect and that their cars, trucks, and planes can't? Men do things to their bodies they would never do to machines, and if they looked at it that way, health might make more sense to them.

Iridology can point the way, but it can't force a man to choose better health. Nor can it be of help when the body has been so long neglected that the point of no return has been reached. Men must come to realize that the functioning, happiness, and stability of their families depend to a large extent on how they take care of themselves. Job performance and successful marriages are directly related to a person's level of health.

As we have mentioned, certain unresolved childhood health problems are often brought into adult life. We need to consider problems and diseases that run in the family. What health problems did our parents have? Do we need to change our food habits to sidestep diseases that run in the family? Or, to overcome the junk food we ate so much of during our teen and early adult years?

The "What's-Wrong-With-Me" Stages of Life

Often, it is when men begin noticing digestive disturbances that they become aware their health is not what it should be. The body is slower in its response. We are not as eager to get going in the morning, and we feel a bit more tired from work when we come home at night. Perhaps there are arguments with the wife—too many of them. Our job may be a source of stress.

Maybe we haven't climbed as far up on the ladder of success as Jones has, when we swore we'd never let him get ahead of us. We're not "keeping up with the Jones'," and it worries us. Financial problems are setting in. So are the aches and pains of the body.

We get acquainted with the doctor at this stage, filling our first prescription. Perhaps tranquilizers for the nerves, or gel for the ulcer. Maybe a diuretic for the kidneys.

Tossing the football to our teenage son, we throw the shoulder out. It's hard to accept that the body isn't what it used to be. The blood pressure is up—not too high yet, but not where it should be either. We make a complete fool of ourself after only three cocktails; the next day we realize we aren't able to hold our liquor as we once did.

Now we reach the compensation stage of life. To cope with the small multiple ills accompanying a so-so level of health that comes directly from our lifestyle, we start contributing to the profits of the local drugstore. We need aspirin for the headaches. Seltzer for the upset stomach. Sleepytime tablets to help get to sleep. Wide-eye tablets to keep us awake and alert on those overtime evenings at work. Laxatives for the bowel. Cold pills. Cough medicine. Chronic disease is well on its way, even though no well-defined symptoms have reared their ugly heads. There is still time to upgrade the health and avoid disease—if the know-how is found.

Next, we reach the "downhill run" stage. Everything is going downhill, but we're too stubborn to do anything about it. The sex life is almost shot. Arguments with the wife escalate. The word "divorce" is popping up. The boss has promoted a man ten years younger than you, and your hair is disappearing fast. We're taking vitamins and protein drinks, but not much good seems to be coming of them. We're getting up three or four times at night to urinate. We feel tired all the time.

The "bottom line" stage is when the doctor tells us the prostate has to be operated on. Or, there's a suspicious-looking tumor in the colon. Or, that you could have a heart attack any day if you don't get that blood pressure down. There are few doctors who can do much for you at this stage, except to help plug the leaks in the lifeboat as they spring, one at a time. By this time, you've worked the thyroid so long, so hard, that the body's recuperative powers are almost negligible.

Ironically, it is at this stage of fully-blown chronic disease that doctors finally know what to do. They have been generally as puzzled as you by the minor, subjective, indefinite feelings of malaise registering off and on for the past ten or twenty years. They can't really cure you even now, but they can give those symptoms of yours a pretty rough time. Surgery may be indicated. Or, your doctor may prescribe a new hotshot drug—one that has powerful side effects.

Of course, there's not all that much time to wait until retirement. Five years. Ten. Then the memory starts to go. We lose the car in the parking lot outside the supermarket, and it takes two hours to find it. Senility? Alzheimer's disease? Will those last years be spent in a rest home?

Ulcers Belong to Executives

It has been said many times, to illustrate the consequences of high-pressure jobs, that a man is working at Ulcers, Inc. He loves his job but he hates the boss, or vice versa. Or, if he is the boss, he has allowed himself to become overwhelmed with facts and decisions requiring creative logic, imagination, memory, thought, precision, and promptness. He has to look into multi-level problems. He has to look for ways out. He has to have it all by five o'clock. This kind of work leads to that early ulcer. All personal considerations have become secondary to the job. His mealtimes are rushed snacks. He goes for a menu that offers the quickest foods (usually prepared a couple of days in advance). He lives on fried foods, quick foods, and his job comes first.

This is the man who has his work in his briefcase so he can pick it up and go—right now. He is well-organized, but to get it to that place, he had to overwork his nervous system and his brain capacity. He is ready to review anything that he has taken up in the last months. He shoulders the troubles and the worries of each day. He often takes on the problems of his employees as well. He does not come home early; he stays in the office, burning the midnight oil. He very seldom takes off a weekend to enjoy himself. He is lost in his job.

If there is a request made, he can never say no. He is always going to take care of it. He has heard that the busy man is always the man who can take care of still more. And if you want anything done, please ask the busiest man to do it. The one who doesn't have much to do doesn't want more. But he is not the executive.

The executive is prepared to respond to any emergency, but when an emergency arises over his health, he cannot do that. He puts off the visit to the doctor.

The executive accepts all invitations. He is made president of the club. He is made advisor, counselor, board member of several organizations. He goes to banquets, eating what is served, even if it is pure poison. He eats at any time of the day, letting his stomach know, "If you are going to live with me, you will have to take it as it comes." He is on every committee possible. He does not sit down and listen to music while he is eating and does not know what it is to relax at a meal. He is always planning for conferences and, at the meal hour, he is talking about the stock market. He is planning for the future.

This sort of person always seems to be reviewing and rethinking those things that did not go so well that morning or the day before. He is ready to set up a new day and a new job plan whenever it is necessary. As far as hobbies are concerned, he knows all about them. He is very clever and can tell you all the things that can be done in an exercise program, but he is always too busy to actually do it. First of all, it is a waste of time and you will find that he cannot stand, sit, or lie down a few moments and do nothing. To take a holiday or weekend and do nothing is something that is just going to mean more work when he gets back. He realizes that he will never get the work done if he does not do some in his spare time.

He may have difficulty delegating work to other people. He finds they are not as efficient as he is, and they do not come through as fast. They are not always good willed. There is animosity, resistance, and resentment. They do not have that self-reliance he can depend on. So, he does it all himself. He carries the whole load—and he can do it for a certain length of time.

Someone like this does not realize that as the nervous system is drained, eventually the physical body is going to rebel. If he has to travel, somebody else has to pick up his bags; he is ready to go and spends no time between planes. He has no time to overcome jet lag. He works all day and drives all night or is on a plane all night. He has to do this to keep the next day's appointments. His appointments are the most important thing in the world. His promises mean something to him and he keeps them. He expects the other person to keep them and when they do not, he lives in disappointment, and it is overdriving all the mental faculties that depletes the powerful executive of all the lovely nerve force he needs in order to keep well. Ulcers usually come from these kinds of activities.

THE ALTERNATIVE

It is tragic that so many Americans do not understand that they don't have to face the so-called "golden years" in a rapidly declining state of health, with virtually nothing to look forward to but operations, pills, and pain.

We can trace the entire course of a chronic disease in the iris, but it does little good unless the patient makes a decision to reverse that course and seek a healthy way of life. Medical science has no "silver bullets" with which to eliminate chronic diseases. You get rid of them or prevent them by working at it.

Hering's law of cure states, "All cure comes from within out, from the head down and in reverse order as the symptoms first appeared." In other words, when we return to a healthy way of life, the body begins retracing, building up strength and throwing off toxic accumulations. We work toward healing crises that generally consist of intense, short-term reversals of old symptoms. When a healing crisis occurs, the body is rejecting old accumulated wastes and toxins. This is Nature's way of keeping the body clean and healthy, and it is the ultimate solution to chronic disease.

Through right nutrition, exercise, fresh air, relaxation, rest, positive attitudes, and an enthusiastic outlook, most people can leave chronic disease behind. The truth about proper nutrition and correct living is no secret. Educating—not medicating—is the way to better health and high-level well-being.

Iridology shows exactly what stages the various tissues and organs of the body are currently in. Most diseases "hide" in the subclinical stage for many years before symptoms manifest, and doctors can't tell what is happening. Iridology can detect these early conditions in time to deal with them nutritionally, with the objective of restoring the body to a right chemical balance. There are mechanical treatments for the mechanical problems like prolapsus, congested lymph glands, anemia of the extremities, and nerve blockages. There are ways of changing attitudes and redirecting the emotions. Women's and men's diseases can be taken care of—by taking the higher path, the way to health through the natural ways we have described.

NATURAL REMEDIES FOR WOMEN'S AND MEN'S DISEASES

Below is a list of some symptoms that men and women experience and the foods that can be used to treat these problems.

Prolapsus of the transverse colon. Slantboard exercises, morning and evening, ten minutes each time. Calcium-rich foods.

Calcium deficiency. Sesame seeds, sunflower seeds, almonds—use nut butters or nut milk drinks daily. Whole cereal grains, kale, barley and kale soup, veal joint broth, milk, cheese, alfalfa tablets, comfrey. Calcium must be taken with vitamins A, D, and C with iodine supplement for best assimilation.

Thyroid problems or iodine deficiency. Nova Scotia dulse, liquid dulse, ocean fish.

Menstrual problems. For suppressed menses, ginger tea. For young girls beginning menses who have missed a period, smart weed tincture. For menstrual hemorrhages, cinnamon tea. For difficult, painful menses with large dark clots, licorice root and black cohosh (tea is best; capsules may be taken if necessary); take a tablespoon of gelatin in juice or water once every four hours, if cramps and heavy clotting persist. A good menstrual tonic is one cup clam nectar, four stalks of celery (chopped finely), pinch of ginger, tablespoon of Whex (dried goat whey), handful of parsley, pinch of red raspberry leaves, fresh chicken bones, pinch of cayenne pepper. Simmer twenty minutes and use broth only. Remember, menstrual blood contains forty times the amount of calcium in the bloodstream, and iron is being lost also. These elements must be replaced.

Anemia (iron deficiency). Liver and other organ meats, eggs, goat milk, green, leafy vegetables, parsley, dandelion root, spirulina, chlorella, bee pollen (teaspoon morning and evening), blackberries and other dark berries, cherries and so forth. Iron is assimilated best if taken with calcium foods and green vegetables or chlorophyll, plus vitamins B-12, C, and A.

Prostate trouble. Zinc, pumpkin seeds, ginseng, vitamin E, sitz baths, pelvis exercises, protomorphogen (if advised by doctor).

Arteriosclerosis. Tissue cleansing, chelation therapy, evening primrose oil, high density lipoproteins, lecithin, B-6, sunflower seeds.

Constipation. All yellow fruits and vegetables are natural laxatives. Eat plenty of fresh, raw fruits and vegetables for the bulk and fiber. Algae seem to have a laxative action, and a teaspoon or two of wheat bran may be taken after meals. I have found that four alfalfa tablets taken after each meal (cracked between the teeth first), help tone the bowel, keep the bowel wall clean, supply iron and trace elements, and feed the beneficial bowel flora. Sodium foods like whey, celery, okra, and green leafy vegetables, help the bowel. Yogurt is excellent for increasing beneficial bowel flora and reducing the putrefactive bacteria.

Maintaining a healthy way of life is a necessity whether you are a man or a woman. Along with nutrition, rest and relaxation are essential to health. Daily exercise is also important in keeping the body healthy.

CHAPTER 12

Hypoglycemia—The Almost Forgotten Disease

Hypoglycemia—low blood sugar—is a condition, like heart disease, that has escalated to epidemic proportions in this century. It is dangerous because the brain, more than any other organ in the body, needs blood sugar to supply its energy needs. Low blood sugar depresses all brain functions which in turn depresses the whole vast array of metabolic processes that take place in the body. Hypoglycemia is accompanied by psychological symptoms as well as physical symptoms, and its effects on the quality of thought, creativity, emotion, and the various other brain centers and activities are pervasive, debilitating, and far-reaching.

The main symptoms are fatigue, weakness, restlessness, irritability, and a sense of general discomfort or uneasiness. Advanced conditions may lead to mental disturbances, delirium, coma, and even death if not taken care of. There are a host of related symptoms and conditions that will be brought out as we go along. Low blood sugar has varied effects, weakening the brain and body functions to such an extent that breakdown in any of the inherently weak organs, tissues, and systems can result, leading to asthma, arthritis, and other conditions.

Since hypoglycemia is, on the surface, the opposite of diabetes (high blood sugar due to lack of sufficient insulin), early medical researchers thought it was a pancreas malfunction in the opposite direction. While it is true that excess insulin can produce low blood sugar, it is also true that other factors can bring about hypoglycemia.

WHAT CAUSES LOW BLOOD SUGAR?

In my experience, chronic disease states can seldom be traced to a single cause. A normal, healthy body eliminates substances that irritate its tissues or cause the low level inflammation that precedes the onset of more serious symptoms. But, if a body is so weakened by deficiencies, poor nutrition, and a high-speed lifestyle that it can't right itself, we are looking at more than a simple malfunction in a single organ.

It is evident that malfunction of the islets of Langerhans in the pancreas can cause diabetes or hypoglycemia, as those who first studied hypoglycemia believed. But, if that is the case, what prevents the body from overcoming this condition? Why does the condition "settle in" and remain? I believe there are other causes and preconditions for hypoglycemia, and we don't have to go far to look for them.

The three greatest enemies to health in our time are white sugar, white flour, and foods cooked in hot grease or oil. White sugar throws the endocrine system out of balance, white flour sticks to the bowel wall and slows elimination, and fried grease disrupts the natural balance of fats needed in the body. Frying destroys lecithin, needed to balance cholesterol and other fats. White sugar depletes vitamins and minerals, especially calcium, which is needed for tissue repair and rebuilding. Americans eat more than 125 pounds of sugar per year. White sugar should be classed as a drug, not a food, because it causes sudden and dramatic changes in the body, depletes valuable nutrients, and has serious undesirable side effects, both short and long term. Our bodies were not designed to handle sugar, and because of the large amount most Americans eat, we should not be suprised to find widespread disturbances in the blood glucose system of the body, as well as other related problems.

The point I want to make here is simple. Once the body's natural defenses are weakened through poor eating and living habits, *any of the inherently weak organs and systems of the body can break down.* Under stress, the weakest link of the chain always breaks first. The same is true of the human body. What causes the blood glucose balance to break down in one person may cause arthritis or heart disease in another.

Whether the pancreas is completely responsible for low blood sugar is another matter. The liver, adrenal glands, thyroid, pituitary, hypothalamus, autonomic nerves, vagus nerve, and intestinal mucosa all play roles in balancing blood sugar.

THE BLOOD SUGAR MAZE

Normally, the body works to keep the blood sugar level at 80-110 mg/100 ml, and hypoglycemia is generally defined as a blood sugar level below 50 mg/100 ml. This definition has proved unworkable because of individual variations in blood sugar and because of the varieties of ways in which low blood sugar affects various individuals.

Let's start with the brain. The appetite center in the hypothalamus most likely monitors blood sugar level and signals the body to eat. Its action is both on the nerves and the glandular system. The sight of food, for example, sends impulses down the vagus nerve to the stomach and starts the digestive juices flowing.

Insulin from the pancreas is secreted as soon as food is in the body. Insulin is the most important hormone in digestion, needed for the tissues to use blood sugar for energy, so the liver can convert extra blood sugar to glycogen for storage, and many other things. The release of insulin can be triggered by glucose (blood sugar), protein, the vagus nerve, glucagon (another secretion of the pancreas), and several other chemicals and processes. Insulin brings the blood sugar down by helping tissues use it and by helping the liver store the excess. We should keep in mind that blood sugar can be made from carbohydrates, protein, or fats, though it is usually taken from carbohydrates. Insulin release can be stopped by epinephrine (adrenaline) or norepinephrine from the adrenal glands or by a signal from the vagus nerve.

Secretion of adrenaline by the adrenals brings up blood sugar in several ways. The adrenals can be signaled by nerves, which is why sudden fear or anger produces almost instant energy. Adrenalin is released into the blood, which causes glycogen to be converted into glucose in the muscles and in the liver, raising the blood sugar and making energy available to the cells.

Glucagon, like insulin, is produced by the pancreas and acts to balance insulin in the blood. The two work together. Glucagon is an extremely powerful chemical, thirty to fifty times as powerful as adrenaline in stimulating glucose production by the liver. Its job is to increase blood sugar, but it is normally closely controlled by a balancing amount of insulin.

Cortisone from the adrenals can convert amino acids to glucose in the liver to raise blood sugar.

Thyroxine, secreted by the thyroid, increases glucose release by the liver (and also increases oxygen uptake so the tissues can turn the glucose into energy). Another thyroid hormone acts to increase blood sugar by magnifying the action of adrenaline and norepinephrine on the liver.

When blood sugar is low, the pituitary releases growth hormone and ACTH. Growth hormone increases blood sugar by blocking its uptake in muscle tissue, while ACTH stimulates the adrenals (which, in turn, stimulate the liver) and acts to convert fats into glucose.

There are several organs, glands, and nerves that influence blood sugar level.

Hypothalamus. Controls appetite, monitors blood sugar, connects with vagus nerve, affects pituitary.

Vagus nerve. Can stimulate digestion and signal adrenals and pancreas to release or stop hormones that raise or lower blood sugar.

Pituitary. Releases growth hormone and ACTH to increase blood sugar; ACTH stimulates adrenals to release cortisone.

Pancreas. Releases insulin to lower blood sugar and glucagon to raise it.

Adrenals. Secrete cortisone, adrenaline, and norepinephrine to increase blood sugar.

Thyroid. Secretes at least two hormones that increase blood sugar level.

Liver. Converts glucose to glycogen with the help of insulin, and glycogen to glucose with the help of adrenaline and many other hormones.

To sum up, we see that hypoglycemia (also diabetes) is primarily a glandular and nerve disorder, with the liver as a key organ for the storage of glycogen and release of glucose through the action of hormones. This is an important factor in how we take care of hypoglycemia.

We should notice that symptoms such as nervousness, heart palpitations, sweating, and hunger, which are common in hypoglycemia, show that the nerves are involved. Symptoms disappear after eating or when adrenaline or other hormones are released.

THE SYMPTOMS OF HYPOGLYCEMIA

Dr. Carlton Frederick has compiled a list of hypoglycemia symptoms from a survey of 2,400 hypoglycemia patients. From the list that follows, he devised a simple test to determine whether you may have hypoglycemia. The test, of course, can't be regarded as conclusive.

To take the test, put a check by the symptoms you experience. Then follow the directions that are below Column 1. If your total is more than 58, you could have hypoglycemia.

More About Symptoms

When hypoglycemia was discovered in 1924 by Dr. Seale Harris, the six-hour glucose tolerance test soon became the primary method of diagnosis. Because some persons showed severe symptoms of hypoglycemia with normal test results and because others "failed" the test, but had no signs of hypoglycemia, the interpretation of the glucose test and consideration of symptoms in diagnosis have been changed.

Symptoms have become very important in understanding hypoglycemia and in taking care of it. Low blood sugar is closely linked with several other conditions.

One doctor, who had symptoms of heart attack, found he had hypoglycemia. He is Dr. Broda Barnes, and he has suggested that hypoglycemia is often accompanied by high blood cholesterol, which could link it to cardiovascular disease.

Allergies can be caused by low blood sugar or aggravated by it. Asthma and hay fever are linked to hypoglycemia, along with frequent colds, flu infections, and fevers. Which one comes first doesn't matter, but we need to recognize that the whole set of respiratory conditions (asthma, bronchitis, etc.) tend to cause adrenal exhaustion, which leads to low blood sugar.

DO YOU HAVE HYPOGLYCEMIA?*

Column 1

☐ Nervousness
☐ Irritability
☐ Depression
☐ Forgetfulness
☐ Insomnia (awakening in the small hours, unable to return to sleep)
☐ Constant worrying
☐ Mental confusion
☐ Antisocial behavior
☐ Unprovoked crying spells
☐ Indecisiveness
☐ Lack of sexual drive (females)
☐ Impotence (males)
☐ Night terrors, nightmares
☐ Phobias, fears
☐ Suicidal thoughts
☐ Restlessness
☐ Nervous breakdowns

Number of checks in
Column 1 multiplied by 3   _ _ _

Number of checks in
Column 2 multiplied by 2   _ _ _

_____

Combined totals of
Columns 1 and 2   _ _ _

Column 2

☐ Exhaustion
☐ Faintness, tremors, cold sweats, weak spells
☐ Vertigo (dizziness or sensations of falling)
☐ Drowsiness
☐ Headaches
☐ Chronic indigestion
☐ A feeling of internal trembling
☐ Palpitation of the heart
☐ Rapid pulse
☐ Muscle pain
☐ Numbness
☐ Allergies
☐ Incoordination
☐ Leg cramps
☐ Blurred vision
☐ Twitching, jerking, cramping of leg muscles
☐ Itching, crawling sensations on skin
☐ Gasping for breath
☐ Smothering spells
☐ Staggering
☐ Episodes of blackout or unconsciousness
☐ Rheumatoid arthritis
☐ Neurodermatitis
☐ Lack of appetite
☐ Compulsive craving for sweets, colas, coffee, tea, chocolate
☐ Joint pains
☐ Abdominal spasms
☐ Obesity
☐ Underweight
☐ Compulsive drinking of alcoholic beverages

*From "Your Meals and Your Arthritis" from *Arthritis: Don't Learn to Live With It* by Carlton Fredericks, ©1981 by Carlton Fredericks.

Dr. S. Gyland has compiled a list of the symptoms of hypoglycemia. The symptoms are listed in order of their frequency in persons who have the disease.

SYMPTOMS OF HYPOGLYCEMIA*

Over 90 Percent

Nervousness

Over 80 Percent

Irritability
Exhaustion
Faintness
Dizziness
Tremors
Cold sweats
Weak spells

Over 70 Percent

Depression
Vertigo
Drowsiness
Headaches

Over 60 Percent

Digestive disturbances
Forgetfulness
Insomnia
Constant worrying
Anxieties

Over 50 Percent

Obesity
Mental confusion
Palpitations
Muscle pain
Indecisiveness
Numbness

Over 40 Percent

Unsocial, asocial, or antisocial
    behavior
Crying spells
Lack of sex drive
Allergies and respiratory problems
Lack of coordination
Leg cramps
Lack of concentration
Blurred vision
Twitching and jerking muscles

Over 30 Percent

Itching and crawling sensations on
    the skin
Gasping for breath
Smothering spells
Staggering
Sighing and yawning

Over 20 Percent

Impotency (males)
Night terrors
Arthritis
Phobias
Fears
Skin conditions
Suicidal impulses
Convulsions

Over 10 Percent

Nervous breakdowns

*Reprinted with the permission of the estate of Dr. S. Gyland.

Arthritis has been associated with low blood sugar. Treatment for hypoglycemia has often resulted in improvement of arthritis symptoms as well.

Anorexia nervosa, an increasing problem with many young women (deliberate starvation), was found to respond well to a special diet regimen designed for hypoglycemics. Dr. Cheryl Hawk treated them with chiropractic, a special diet, and vitamin and mineral supplements.

Alcoholism and liver disease are nearly always found to produce hypoglycemia. In many cases, the urge to drink has come from low blood sugar, and desire for alcohol stops as special dieting counteracts the blood sugar problem. In this case, either alcoholism or hypoglycemia can produce the other.

Sluggish liver, according to Dr. Broda Barnes, is the main functional disability in hypoglycemia, but he suggests this is always due to hypothyroidism. Dr. Barnes believes that all hypoglycemia, and disease conditions that follow or accompany it, are most likely secondary results of hypothyroidism.

WHAT EXPERIMENTS REVEAL

Experiments have given us valuable information about blood sugar levels.

When healthy persons fasted to the point of starvation, their glucose blood levels did not drop to the hypoglycemic level—below 50 mg/100 ml.

- Insulin injected into the blood causes an almost immediate hypoglycemic reaction. Subjects of such experiments feel tired, depressed, hungry, nervous, and irritable. Some have shown anger and rage to the point where they had to be given fruit juice to restore emotional equilibrium.
- Hypoglycemia is common in hepatitis and cirrhosis victims as well as in alcoholics. Liver damage is obviously one source of hypoglycemia. Heavy metal poisoning, which damages the liver, also produces it.
- Toxic thyroid cases are generally hypoglycemia. Hypothyroidism has been connected with low blood sugar by Dr. Broda Barnes, who has treated thousands of cases of hypothyroidism. He has not found hypoglycemia in any of his patients taking thyroid hormone to raise the level of thyroid function.
- Removal of the pituitary gland in laboratory animals resulted in extreme sensitivity to insulin and in hypoglycemia.
- Kidney failure with excessive excretion of glucose has produced hypoglycemia.
- Dr. Harvey M. Ross and Jeraldine Saunders, authors of *Hypoglycemia: The Disease Your Doctor Won't Treat*, estimate that

over 50 percent of the American people have hypoglycemia. More conservative estimates give us a figure of around 50 million persons in this country.

- Experiments have shown that deficiencies in pantothenic acid and vitamin C caused disruption in corticosteroid production and, later, symptoms of adrenal exhaustion. This can obviously lead to hypoglycemia.
- Dr. William Philpot has found hypoglycemic responses in individuals to pasteurized cow's milk, cream cheese, hydrocarbons, and other noncarbohydrates. This appears to be more of an allergic reaction than anything else. He found that this was a highly specific response by certain people to certain substances.
- When adrenal secretions were blocked in laboratory animals, a tiny dose of insulin would cause hypoglycemia. Normally functioning animals had no response to the same size dose.
- Dr. E.M. Abrahamson has shown that serious mental problems are often accompanied by hypoglycemia. There is no proof, however, that these problems were caused by hypoglycemia.
- Extracts from the pituitary glands of slaughterhouse animals, if injected into normal animals, stimulate increased blood sugar. The pituitary secretes hormones that cause the thyroid and adrenals to release certain hormones of their own which influence blood sugar levels.
- Injection of adrenal extracts into animals caused blood sugar to rise to the point where it was being excreted in the urine.

TAKING CARE OF HYPOGLYCEMIA

In taking care of hypoglycemia, the wholistic procedure of building up the body, mind, and spirit should be followed.

First, we consider the brain, glands, nerves, and mental aspects. Because hypoglycemia results in fatigue, depression, and restlessness, we encourage a positive attitude, rest, peaceful activities, and avoidance of anything stressful, emphasizing that proper foods will soon improve the physical and biochemical problems. We must bring the brain foods into the diet—animal proteins, eggs, nuts, and seeds in the form of nut and seed milk drinks or butters, cod fish roe, cheese, and so on. We eliminate sugar, coffee, tea, alcohol, sweets, white bread, and other white flour products. Head lettuce and orange juice are out, along with fried foods. All meat should be roasted, broiled, or prepared in soups or stews. Vegetables—plenty of fresh, raw vegetables—will help provide the glucose the body needs, especially the brain. We recall that what feeds the brain also feeds the nerves and glands. It would be wise to cut down on fruit from the supermarket, using discretion to avoid fruits that have been picked before they are ripe.

Instead of two or three meals a day, we should have smaller meals—especially the last meal in the day—and have five or six. Or, we can call the meals "meals," and the in-between eating, "snacks." The idea is to eat small servings of protein at least four of the five or six times.

Now, when I say the brain is a phosphorus organ, I mean we must have the high-quality lecithin and nerve fats in our foods to provide the highly-evolved phosphorus. Eggs, boiled or poached; cod fish roe added to tomato juice, sesame seed butter, and so forth, should be taken.

The pancreas, particularly the islets of Langerhans and the insulin made there, need zinc and sulphur foods. The liver can be detoxified and rejuvenated with chlorophyll, aloe vera, and the high iron foods. The raw vegetables and chlorophyll will help cleanse the liver, while the protein and iron foods will build it up. Calcium, "the knitter," is important in tissue restoration as well, and we get it from the nuts and seeds that provide some of our lecithin and high-quality lipids, and from cod fish roe. We can have some raw goat milk, too.

In the case of the adrenals, vitamin C is especially important, and we must have plenty of it. For the thyroid, take Nova Scotia dulse to supply iodine.

There are times when we should use vitamin and mineral supplements, although I believe that we should get most of our chemical elements from foods. Table 12.1 outlines a program of vitamin supplements for hypoglycemics. The supplements shown in the Table should be taken three times a day, before meals.

Table 12.1   Vitamin Program for Hypoglycemics

Vitamin	Recommended Amount
Vitamin A	25,000 I.U.
Vitamin B-1	10 mg
Vitamin B-2	10 mg
Vitamin B-3	100 mg
Vitamin B-6	50 mg
Vitamin B-12	50 mg
Niacin	50 mg
Pantothenic acid	100 mg
Folic acid	80 mcg
Vitamin C	1 gm
Bioflavinoids	350 mg
Vitamin E	100 I.U.
Choline	300 mg
Inositol	90 mg

It is possible that mechanical manipulation such as chiropractic and massage can help with the nerve supply and relaxation. We realize that stress is a major factor in hypoglycemia. Slant board exercises should be considered to move the blood to the head, and it would be good to include the bouncer exercises, twice a day for ten minutes at a time.

SUMMARY

Hypoglycemia appears to be primarily a glandular disorder produced by excessive use of white sugar and other foodless foods, along with stress and hypoactive liver. It is best taken care of by relaxation, rest, a high protein diet, and avoidance of conflict and stress. Foods that are good for the hypoglycemic person are those that are high in animal lecithin (phospholipids) for the brain and glands; calcium for the nerves and tissue rejuvenation; iron for the liver; zinc for the pancreas; sulphur for the brain and pancreas; and vitamins as necessary to supplement the diet.

PART THREE
Building Health Naturally

CHAPTER 13
Communication With Our Bodies

As we consider how our body works, the first thing we should realize is that our occupation and marriage affect us physically. Stress comes from all areas of life, and tension and discontent can make us ill.

In considering our job, we have to decide whether we are a square peg in a round hole or a round peg in a round hole. Are we suited to the job we have? Are we using our talents? Most people love some aspects of their job and hate others. Perhaps our lifestyle could be changed so that we derive more satisfaction from our daily routine.

We must carefully consider whether the symptoms our bodies reveal to us are "messages" telling us that something we are doing is harmful, or whether these symptoms have developed from causes that are unrelated to external events. In his classic book *The Stress of Life,* Hans Selye showed us how many different physical symptoms can be traced to stress. He considered stress to be a common and largely overlooked contributing factor to many diseases, including heart disease, cancer, and gastrointestinal problems like ulcers or colitis. When symptoms appear, then, it becomes very important to ask ourselves, "Is my body trying to communicate something to me about my way of living? My attitude? My relationships? My emotional responses to events and tasks in my job or profession?"

One of my patients had a serious liver ailment. He had been working in accounting for twelve years and didn't like it. I spoke to him about the possible relationship between his health and his job. He said that he liked people and wished he could work more with people, but he had seven children, so he felt it was more important to keep his job. He didn't feel he had the courage to go out and look for work that he truly liked, but I encouraged him and gave him dietary counsel that would be of some help.

After taking a three-month sabbatical, he found a job that enabled him to work with people, and now he makes more money and is a more successful, harmonious, and joyous person. His liver condition cleared up completely!

In this story is a lesson. It is claimed that 90 percent of the people today are misfits in their jobs. Employers have something to complain about, if this is true. Misfits goof off and waste hours because they can't concentrate, don't like the job, and are clock watchers. They are ready to leave the moment it is quitting time.

Job dissatisfaction is a major source of stress, and stress dramatically increases the body's rate of utilization of the chemical elements, vitamins, enzymes, and other substances important to metabolism. Depletion of these metabolically important biochemicals weakens the body's defenses against disease by altering body chemistry in subtle and not-so-subtle ways. Of course, similar deficiencies can be caused by an imbalanced or inadequate diet, by drug abuse, and by habits like overwork or chronic lack of sufficient sleep.

People should be working in jobs where their abilities and talents can be used, or they may become frustrated, unhappy and, consequently, deficient in the chemical elements needed to sustain life. Expression of natural gifts and abilities in our professions may be more important to health than most people realize. Frustration and unhappiness lead to chemical deficiencies which, in turn, lead to diseases of many kinds.

For example, some people are esthetically inclined, and sensitive. They may love music or art. I have found that such people may lose their health if they are cut off from the things in life that are dear to them. They need to be around the music or art that they love to feel good about themselves and to digest their foods properly.

DEFICIENCY SYMPTOMS

In order to be happy, we should not only be satisfied with what we are doing; it is also important to eat the right foods to have the proper chemical elements in the body. When the body lacks specific chemical elements, certain conditions are produced. We should know more about these conditions.

Magnesium

One condition we should know about is magnesium deficiency. The pain that could be a symptom of this deficiency will be worse when a person is sitting still, and will be even more severe at night.

When a person cannot bear to be touched or when the pain runs from above to below, magnesium is needed. Perspiration may be burning and profuse, a wave like warm water seems to pass through the body (associated with shivers down the spine), hot, muggy weather is unbearable, and the mind and senses are dull in the open air. Food aggravates the magnesium-deficient person, drink produces toothache, a rushing sound is heard, and the area between the toes is raw and the knees are weak.

Iodine

Symptoms of iodine deficiency are goiter, doughy skin, and chronic low energy or fatigue. Other symptoms include frothy salivation, running saliva, palpitations at high altitudes, and short, labored breathing. The urine may be cloudy and have a strong odor and earth-like sediment. Iodine deficiency may be indicated by throbbing arteries, difficulty in swallowing food, unilateral ailments (worse on the left side), numb fingers, occasional prostration, trouble with the throat, restless eyes, constant tiredness and shyness, tonsil trouble, a fluttering sound in the ears, catarrh, popping of the underjaw, and clenching of the jaws.

Potassium

Potassium phosphate is needed by the entire muscular system, both the voluntary and involuntary muscles, as well as all muscular fibers and cells throughout the body. Potassium plays an important part in the synthetic processes of the chemical combination of organic life, in the formation of glycogen from glucose, in the digestion and assimilation of fats and proteins, in the manufacture of red blood cells, in brain functioning, and in the normal processes of the heart and liver.

Potassium deficiency symptoms may include muscle weakness, cramps, spasms, heart palpitations, fatigue, irritability, swollen lymph glands, painful menses, irritated throat and nasal passages, and frequent colds. Because the potassium-deficient individual will have an over-acidic body chemistry (due to insufficient neutralization of metabolic acids when potassium is insufficient), arthritic symptoms may appear and any previously existing arthritis condition will be aggravated. The temper may be short and aggravations may be many due to irritated nerves. Oxygenation of the brain and tissues, which requires potassium, is reduced, resulting in less efficient mental functioning and lowered muscle strength and tone. Fermentation in the bowel, excessive gas formation, and abdominal discomfort may be present, since there is not enough potassium to neutralize bowel acids. Skin eruptions may increase. Earaches, fevers, diarrhea, dizziness, excessive sleepiness, shallow breathing, and indigestion are common potassium deficiency symptoms.

Mental symptoms of potassium deficiency frequently include unreasonable fears, poor memory, anxiety, antagonism, loss of motivation, noise intolerance, slurred speech, and inability to function in any challenging job or social environment requiring quick physical or mental responses.

Sodium

There is a definite connection between the chemical elements and the symptoms we read in the iris. With this reading, we can see just where the chemical is needed. Sodium gives such definite symptoms that they are very useful to know. It is one of the most important health-supportive elements.

Sodium is active in the lymph and blood. Food sodium, iron, and chlorine make the blood what it is—a salty liquid. Sodium is needed to keep calcium and magnesium dissolved in the blood. Lack of sodium is often followed by calcium deposits in joints, joint stiffness, rheumatism, gout, gallstones, and other ailments. It helps prevent excess or undesirable blood clots, which could cause strokes, paralysis, thrombosis, and other problems. Food sodium helps keep milk protein in solution. It plays an important part in salivation, bile action, pancreatic functioning, and the emulsification of fat. The deficiency of sodium results in gas generation, bloating, and constipation.

Sodium is found in the secretory glands, the synovial, the serous membranes, and the throat and alimentary canal. It helps increase osmosis and keeps whole calcium in solution. It helps control albumen and fibrin and keep it in solution, and is essential for the spleen, which is a sodium organ.

Calcium

We seem to be going calcium crazy in this country at the present time. Calcium is of greatest importance in the growth of a baby and in controlling bleeding tendencies. Adequate calcium is necessary to help prevent rickets, tuberculosis, bone softening, and osteoporosis. But it is *food calcium* that we need, not inorganic calcium salts such as those that are found in the drug or health food stores. Calcium cannot be utilized properly by the body unless it is accompanied by magnesium, phosphorus, and vitamins A, D, and C. This occurs normally only in foods. If necessary, bone meal may be taken as a balanced source of most of these ingredients.

Calcium deficiency symptoms usually start with muscle discomfort—cramps, numbness, and tingling in the arms and legs. Long-term calcium deficiency in children causes rickets and stunted growth, and osteoporosis in adults (particularly post-menopausal women). Osteoporosis is a disease in which bone porosity greatly increases fragility and danger of bone breakage, particularly in the elderly. Osteomalacia, another adult calcium-deficiency condition, results in bone softening.

Joint pains, heart palpitations, dental caries, insomnia, slow pulse rate, and slow blood clotting all may indicate calcium deficiency. Also, symptoms claimed to be associated with aging—such as backaches, tremors of the hands, difficulty in sleeping, and deep bone pains—are more likely to be caused by calcium deficiency.

Calcium deficiency, like that of potassium, may result in impaired memory, poor thinking, and mental fatigue. All normal functions and responses take place slowly and with some difficulty. An individual with this deficiency will be impatient, insensitive, indifferent to the needs and problems of others, and indifferent to the beauty and joy in life. He may be selfish, antisocial, bad-tempered, moody, accident-prone, depressed, suspicious, and distrustful.

I also believe that a deficiency of calcium may contribute to sinus problems, bronchitis, colds, ulcers, eczema, asthma, hemorrhoids, varicose veins, anemia, rheumatism, and heart problems.

Silicon

Silicon is needed by the brain, nerves, glands, skin, hair, and nails. Possibly the first symptom of silicon deficiency is lack of sheen in the hair or nails, or the appearance of dandruff. Other symptoms soon follow.

A silicon-deficient person is abnormally sensitive to light, sounds, being touched, and pain. The lips and skin become dry, and scabs may form behind the ears. The nose, eyes, ears, and anus may itch. Cuts become easily and quickly infected. Bronchial infections are frequent, tendons are tender, and muscle coordination is impaired. There may be sores on the lips, or painful gums. Gout pain is intensified by lack of silicon.

Psychological symptoms of silicon deficiency include weeping spells, mood swings, and a tendency to hypochondria and morbid thoughts. Optimism in the morning shades into depression in the evening. The person's disposition may vacillate between submissiveness and willful rebellion, between obedience and disobedience, agreement and whimsical opposition to everything, cowardice and aggressive behavior. Chronic silicon deficiency is often associated with lung disease such as tuberculosis.

Other Deficiency Symptoms

The list below shows symptoms and the minerals and elements used to treat these symptoms. These are some of the most common conditions my patients have.

Acidosis: Depletion of the alkali reserves of the body. Need Sodium, Potassium, Calcium, Magnesium.
Acne: Eczema, muddy skin, pimples. Need Chlorine, Sulphur, Iodine, Iron and Copper, Hydrogen, Silicon.
Anemia: Malnutrition, underweight. Need Nitrogen, Calcium, Phosphorus, Iron, Copper, Manganese.

Arthritis: Rheumatism, gout. Need Sodium, Iodine, Magnesium, Hydrogen, and Sulphur.

Asthma: Need Iron, Copper and Manganese, Oxygen, Hydrogen.

Autointoxication: (Absorption of impurities) Chlorine, Potassium, Sodium, Iodine, Calcium, Silicon.

Biliousness: Need Sodium, Chlorine, Potassium, Silicon.

Blood pressure: (High) Need Sodium, Hydrogen, Magnesium, and Potassium.

Boils: Need Silicon, Chlorine, Sulphur.

Bright's disease: Need Sodium, Hydrogen, Potassium, Magnesium, and Oxygen.

Bronchitis: Colds, sinus trouble, catarrh. Need Iron, Copper, Manganese, Oxygen, Hydrogen, Calcium, Silicon.

Colitis: Mucus, hyperacidity, ulcer of digestive organs, gastric and duodenal enteritis, gastritis.

Constipation: Need Sodium, Magnesium, Chlorine, Hydrogen.

Diabetic people: Need Sodium.

Eyesight failing: Cataract. Need Fluorine, Silicon, Phosphorus.

Falling hair: Need Sulphur, Silicon, Fluorine, Calcium, Phosphorus, Iodine.

Fingernails: Thin, hard, brittle. Need Calcium, Manganese, Fluorine.

Gallbladder disorders, gallstones: Jaundice. Need Sodium, Chlorine, Magnesium, Hydrogen.

Goiter: Simple. Need Iodine, Iron, Manganese, Calcium, Sodium, Phosphorus, Chlorine.

Hardening of the arteries: Need Potassium, Hydrogen, Magnesium.

Hay fever: Need Calcium, Potassium, Phosphorus.

Leucorrhea: Need Calcium, Phosphorus.

Low vitality: No endurance, "lack of pep." Need Nitrogen, Sodium, Potassium.

Nervousness: Neuralgia, nerve exhaustion. Calcium, Phosphorus, Nitrogen, Iron, Copper, Manganese.

Obesity: Reducing. Need Silicon, Chlorine, Iodine, Potassium.

Prostate gland enlargement: Need Iron, Copper, Manganese, and Calcium.

Poor Circulation: Need Calcium, Phosphorus, Iron, Magnesium.

Sex indifference: Need Phosphorus, Iron, Copper, Sulphur, Manganese, Nitrogen.

Teeth and Gums: Teeth decay, spongy and bleeding gums. Need Calcium, Phosphorus, Silicon, Fluorine, Nitrogen.

Tuberculosis: Need Nitrogen, Calcium, Phosphorus, Silicon, Oxygen, Fluorine, Iron, Copper, and Manganese.

Undernourished children: Need Calcium, Phosphorus, Iodine, Iron, and Magnesium.

Table 13.1, The Iridology Nutrition Chart, tells more about the chemicals needed by each organ. It also lists the foods that provide these chemicals.

Table 13.1   Iridology Nutrition Chart

Organ	Vitamin	Mineral	Food Source
ADRENALS	C,E,F, Pantothenic acid	Calcium, Sodium,Fluorine, Iodine, Iron, Magnesium, Manganese, Silicon, Sulphur, Tin, Zinc	Juniper, Licorice Root, Blood Root, Gota Kola, Borage, Ginseng, Kelp, Parsley
BLADDER	A,D	Manganese, Potassium	Comfrey, Cornsilk, Golden Seal, Oat Straw, Uva ursi, Yarrow
BONES/JOINTS	A,B1,C,D, Folic Acid	Calcium, Phosphorus,Fluorine, Potassium, Silicon, Sodium, Sulphur	Dandelion Root
BRAIN	B Complex, B12,C,D,E,G	Calcium, Copper, Fluorine, Iodine, Iron, Magnesium, Manganese, Phosphorus, Silicon, Sulphur	Gota Kola, Oat Straw, Red Clover, Valerian, Orange Blossom, Ginseng, Rosemary, Rue Sage, St. Johnswort, Walnuts
CIRCULATION/BLOOD VESSEL	A,B,B1,C,D,G,Niacin	Magnesium, Phosphorus, Silicon, Fluorine, Iodine, Iron, Manganese, Sulphur	Hawthorne berry tea, Oat Straw tea, Sprouts, Prickly Nettle, Cayenne
COLON	A,C,D,F	Sodium, Potassium, Magnesium, Iron	Flaxseed,Psyllium seed, Slippery Elm, Alfalfa, Comfrey Root, Chlorophyll
EARS	A,B,C,D	Potassium, Calcium, Phosphorus	Garlic, Hyssop/Sage combination, Malv flowers, Mullein, Shavegrass, Yellow doc
EYES	A,B2,C	Calcium, Silicon, Sodium, Fluorine, Manganese, Sulphur	Eyebright, Oat Straw, Dandelion Root, Camomile, Golden Seal, Marshmallow, Raspberry, Rose petals
GALL BLADDER	A,C,E	Iodine, Sulphur, Chlorine, Iron, Potassium, Sodium	Dandelion, Boldo, Cascara sagrada, Chicory, Golden Seal, Marigold, Rosemary, Yellow Dock, Comfrey
HEART	A,B,B1,C,D,E	Calcium, Iron, Magnesium, Manganese, Nitrogen, Phosphorus, Potassium, Silicon	Hawthorn berry, Anise seed, Cayenne, Garlic, Horehound, Mistletoe
KIDNEYS	A, B12,C,E	Potassium, Chlorine, Iron, Manganese, Magnesium	Alfalfa, Uva ursi, Blood Root, Buchu, Comfrey, Juniper, Oat Straw, Parsley, Scurvygrass, Shavegrass
LIVER	A,B12,C,E, Niacin	Iron, Potassium, Chlorine, Copper, Iodine, Magnesium, Sodium	Yellowdock, Alfalfa seeds, Archangelica, Artichoke, Blue violet, Boldo, Cascara sagrada, Dandelion, Golden Seal, Marigold, Mullein, Nettle, Oat Straw, Saw palmetto, White oak bark
LUNGS/BRONCHIALS	A,B,C,D	Calcium, Copper, Fluorine, Iron, Oxygen, Silicon	Comfrey, Lungwort, Angelica, Elecampane, Eucalyptus, Fenugreek, Licorice, Marshmallow, Mullein, Sage, Thyme
LYMPH SYSTEM	B Complex,E	Potassium, Sodium,Chlorine	Pokeweed, Dandelion Root, Golden Seal, Cascara sagrada, Blue violet tea
MAMMARY GLAND	A,B1	Chlorine, Sodium, Potassium	Anise seed, Black Cohosh, Fennel, Mullein
MEDULLA	C,B Complex	Phosphorus, Silicon, Sulphur	Sage, Rue
MOUTH/THROAT	A,B,C,D	Iodine	Comfrey, Fenugreek, Golden Seal, Licorice, Raspberry, Sage
MUSCLES	A,B1,B6,C,D,E,G	Nitrogen, Potassium,Chlorine, Iron, Sodium	Rye, Bananas
NAILS	A,D	Calcium, Silicon, Phosphorus, Potassium, Sodium, Sulphur	Oat Straw
NERVES	A,B Complex,B1,B2,B6, Niacin, C,D,G	Phosphorus, Calcium, Sulphur, Iodine, Magnesium, Manganese	Oat Straw, Valerian, Balm, Lavender, Orange blossoms, Passion flower, Peppermint
NOSE/SINUS	A,C,D	Calcium, Chlorine, Silicon	Licorice, Comfrey, Eucalyptus, Fenugreek Golden Seal, Mint, Sage

Table 13.1—*Continued*

Organ	Vitamin	Mineral	Food Source
OVARIES/GONADS	A,B,B12,C,E,F	Calcium, Zinc, Fluorine, Iodine, Iron, Phosphorus, Silicon	Elderberry, Raspberry, Black Cohosh (ovaries), Catnip, Damiana (testes)
PANCREAS	B Complex, B1,B12	Sodium, Chlorine, Copper, Iron, Magnesium, Potassium, Silicon, Zinc	Dandelion, Alfalfa, Beanpods, Eucalyptus, Goldenrod, Juniperberry
PINEAL/PITUITARY	B Complex,E	Bromine, Iodine, Manganese, Phosphorus, Silicon, Sulphur	Mistletoe, Sage, Veronica
PROSTATE	C,B,B12,E,F	Zinc, Calcium, Fluorine, Iron, Potassium, Silicon, Sulphur	Golden Seal, Juniperberry, Buchu, Gota Kola, Kelp, Uva ursi
SPLEEN	C,B Complex	Copper, Iron, Chlorine, Fluorine, Magnesium, Potassium, Sodium	Dandelion Root, Cascara sagrada, Chaparral, Pokeweed
SPINE	A,B,C,D	Calcium, Sodium, Silicon	Comfrey, Barley, Dandelion
SKIN	A,B1,B2,C,G, Niacin, PABA	Silicon, Copper, Iron, Manganese, Potassium, Sodium, Sulphur	Oat Straw, Alfalfa, Bay leaf, Burdock, Chickweed, Elderflower, Sarsaparilla, Yarrow
STOMACH	A,B1,B2,C,D,G, Folic Acid, Niacin	Chlorine, Iron, Magnesium, Potassium, Sodium, Sulphur	Comfrey, Fenugreek, Peppermint, Archangelica, Ginger, Papaya, Raspberry, Slippery Elm, Alfalfa
THYMUS	B	Calcium, Fluorine, Iron, Silicon	Dandelion Root
THYROID	A,B6,B12,C,D,E	Iodine, Chlorine, Magnesium, Potassium, Sodium	Dulse, Horseradish, Parsley, Pokeweed (black), Radish, Kelp
TEETH/GUMS	A,B2,C,D	Calcium, Sodium, Silicon,Fluorine, Phosphorus, Sulphur	Ginger, Myrrh, Shepherd's Purse, Tormentilla, Walnut leaves
UTERUS	B Complex,B12,C,E,F	Calcium, Silicon, Zinc	Black Cohosh, Red Raspberries, Rue

THE IRIDOLOGY CONNECTION

When our bodies are communicating to us that something is wrong, it is good to know that the iridologist will know how to find out what it is and what chemical elements we need. When the body breaks down, and subacute, chronic, and degenerative conditions appear, more calcium, sodium, and potassium are needed to liquefy the mucus congestion in the tissues that accompanies these chronic conditions. In fact, by using iridology we can tell when an acute, subacute, chronic, or degenerative condition exists in the body, where it exists, and whether it is being successfully reversed by a particular health regimen. We can retrace and clear up dry catarrhal conditions that settle in various organs in the form of phlegm and mucus. Liquefying and breaking down catarrhal congestion takes place in the lung structure as well as in other parts of the body.

Catarrh comes from the Greek words meaning "flow down." These old chronic conditions must be brought to a flowing stage again. The iridologist can monitor our condition while this is happening, and will be able to see when the reversal process is complete. Then, he can put us on the road to health.

THE REVERSAL PROCESS

In the reversal process, dried tissue settlement will be liquefied and a running process will be stimulated. The nose and ears will run, and there may be discharges from the vaginal tract and other body orifices. A cold could appear in the bursae of the shoulder, and during the reversal process the old aches and pains from the past may appear because chronic, hardened toxic settlements are in the body and have participated in the development of chronic disease. The reversal process will bring these conditions into a liquefied state, a running state, and this eventually will bring a patient back to health.

What a wonderful opportunity we have in iridology—to recognize the need for chemical elements and to be able to evaluate the success or failure of a diet program by looking at the iris!

When we are taking care of the organs in the body, we do not think in terms of treating disease. We are awakening, quickening, and bringing the functioning ability of an organ up to normal. When we do this, that organ becomes sufficiently stimulated to begin eliminating toxic settlements that have accumulated over the years. The elimination of stored toxic settlements restores youthfulness in that tissue, and youthfulness is sustained by eating plenty of sodium foods.

In order for the iridologist to see healing signs in the iris, he has to recognize the importance of sodium and calcium for the reversal process. Our lymph and blood need sodium for cleansing, energy, and power. All the body functions need calcium. Without it, we cannot reverse an abnormal health condition. We need calcium for vitality and endurance. By the symptoms presented to us, the body communicates its needs for certain chemical elements. Symptoms always communicate needs.

When the reversal process is successfully completed, symptoms will disappear. That doesn't mean that tissue integrity is completely restored in the body, but it does mean that the right things are being done and that tissue correction is taking place. Usually, at least a year is required for any chronic condition or any ailment that has existed for many years to be reversed. Iridology is the only analysis I know of that will show when the reversal process has accomplished tissue correction in the body.

As I have said before, iridology does not treat disease. It deals with organ function. The iridologist is interested in chemical and mineral deficiency and in restoring chemical balance. In restoring this balance, he can send the patient in the right direction. The body starts to recuperate.

IRIDOLOGY AND THE OTHER HEALING ARTS

Iridology can be combined with the other drugless healing arts and enhances each of them. The iridologist can work with the health practitioner, whether he be an acupuncturist, homeopath, herbalist, chiropractor, or other practitioner. Working together, they can bring the patient to the point of optimum health.

Herbology

The iridologist can work with the herbalist. There are conditions in all parts of the body that respond very well to certain herbs.

The late John Christopher, possibly the most outstanding herbalist in this century, always took a teaspoon of red cayenne pepper before every lecture. His bright red complexion was a common topic of conversation among his students, but he had a good reason for taking it. The cayenne pepper increased the circulation in the extremities that was so necessary to get the brain working at full efficiency.

Herbal treatments are often effective in removing symptoms and restoring well-being, as iridology shows. We need to understand this kind of communication. When we are well, our body is signaling that everything is great.

Homeopathy

Homeopathy is a wonderful health art. It deals with the chemical elements in the body and uses the twelve tissue salts to supply the need for certain amounts of sulphur, calcium, magnesium, and other elements to take care of the deficiencies in the body. (See Chapter 16 for more on homeopathy.)

Today, many homeopaths use iridology. Ignatz Von Peczely, the founder of iridology, did wonderful things using iridology and homeopathic remedies. He cured many patients, and it is said that he was paid well enough to put twelve medical students through school.

Like many practitioners in the health arts, homeopaths find that iridology is very useful in monitoring the health of their patients. With iridology, the homeopath can closely watch the effectiveness of the cell salts they have advised their patients to use.

Chiropractic

There is no reason why we should not use diet and iridology along with chiropractic. If there is inherent weaknesses in the spinal area, who will know except the iridologist? Chiropractic methods do not reveal inherent weaknesses apart from the use of iridology. Yet, scoliosis, lordosis, and other abnormal spinal conditions commonly treated by chiropractic are related to our inherent weaknesses. When a chiropractor uses iridology to identify inherent weakness in the spinal vertebra, he knows that a chiropractic treatment will not solve the problem unless used together with calcium foods or calcium supplementation. It would be a wonderful thing to be able to quicken all the organs and supply all the food elements to provide the nerve supply to every organ and allow our bodies to function properly.

FATHER KNEIPP

Father Kneipp is an example of someone who listened to what his body was telling him and attempted to find a cure for his ailment.

Father Sebastian Kneipp was born in Bavaria in 1821. Given up to die from tuberculosis at the age of 26, he cured himself by walking in the snow and taking daily cold water baths. He became a well-known advocate of cold water baths and herbal teas.

Father Kneipp built a sanitarium at Worishofen, Germany, where he treated as many as 4,000 patients weekly during the later years of the nineteenth century. He believed cold water is live water, while hot water is dead water. Photos in his book, *My Water Cure*, show long lines of people wading knee deep in his cold water baths and walking around, letting the air dry their legs, as he instructed.

Juniper berry tea was one of his favorites for stimulating circulation of the blood. He recommended many other herbal teas for various conditions.

Using herbal therapy and water treatments, Father Kneipp helped many people. He treated princes, popes, and all kinds of men who came to him for a program for wellness.

When we go over the biographies of famous men in the healing arts, we almost come to believe that each sufferer has to learn to cure himself. Where is the man who knows all these wholistic arts and who can look at all your symptoms and say, "You need silicon for skin problems, calcium for bone troubles, sodium for an acid stomach, bad spleen, and congested lymph system?" You'll have to go to an iridologist to find out.

How many doctors know the communication that is necessary in this body, and how to manage their patients' physical, mental, and spiritual needs? No one man can know all these things. It requires a lifetime of study. We should be students all our lives, and be able to cooperate with doctors who have an art of healing that is more advanced or different from ours.

NUTRITION IS ESSENTIAL

Once we have sensed that something is wrong in our bodies and have consulted an iridologist, we must follow his instructions and the diet he has planned. A person cannot get well without diet.

Sodium is one of the most important elements our bodies need, and it is often lacking. If you are a vegetarian and live on greens that are full of potassium, you may need more sodium. All people should increase the sodium supply in the body by eating foods that are rich in sodium. Both hot and cold climates use up sodium salts. Being in love makes the assimilation of sodium salts easier and more efficient. Positive emotions assist in more rapid assimilation and utilization of sodium. Under unfavorable emotions or passions, sodium salts are excreted in the urine. A loving state of mind is favorable to health. Bad temper, excitement, jealousy, envy, hate, and melancholy always have an unfavorable effect on the chemistry of the body or upon health. The doctor must know a great deal about how our bodies communicate their needs to us in order to be effective in this work with patients.

RESTORING DEFICIENCIES

When a person suffers from flu, pneumonia, or lung ailments, salts are precipitated into the urine. In such cases, the lost salts must be resupplied first, and the other elements will be taken care of later. These ailments can usually be cured by sodium foods, unless the disease has progressed to such an extent that food alone will not reverse it. Of course, a balanced diet is needed along with the sodium foods.

Many people ask me what diet is helpful for high blood pressure. We have to first determine the cause of the high blood pressure. High blood pressure is a symptom, and the cause should be removed. It could be caused by poor circulation, anemic conditions, or dysfunction of the heart. Once the cause is cared for, the necessary diet can be supplied.

NUTRITION ISN'T EVERYTHING

People use diets for all kinds of conditions. Sometimes, however, other treatments must be used, along with diet. The retroversion of the uterus or prolapsus of the colon are examples of conditions that require additional treatment.

All of the drugless treatments in the healing arts are useful for correcting certain health conditions, considering the great variety of health problems that exist. But none of the treatments will work without foods to build new tissue in place of old. Putting in new tissue and replacing the old tissue is what I call "correction therapy."

Some people in the health arts recommend breathing exercises, but these exercises must be combined with a diet of iron-rich foods, which increase the oxygen-carrying capacity of the blood. We can increase oxygen in our bodies by walking in fresh air up in the hills and follow this up by including iron-rich foods in our diet.

The red corpuscles of the blood are manufactured in the body more slowly in some people than others. It is difficult to tell how long a red cell lasts or works in the body, but it is usually about 120 days. These cells are manufactured utilizing the iron derived from the food we eat. They are manufactured rapidly in high altitudes where less oxygen is in the air, and more red blood cells are needed to attract it in the lungs. They are also manufactured more rapidly during love states, as may be determined in the laboratory.

THE BODY'S DEFENSES

The human system is like a battlefield. An amazing army of bacteria and viruses are always trying to get into the body, and many succeed. There is a greater battle going on in the body than was carried on in the last world war!

Millions of bacteria are at work. Chlorine, sulphur, flourine, magnesium, sodium, and potassium are weapons that work for health. Each element has a role in controlling or eliminating unwanted bacteria and viruses from our bodies. Chlorine and fluorine are powerful germicidal agents. We need them and other chemical elements for our bodies to work properly. Our immunity from disease is dependent in part upon our reserve of these chemical elements.

When we understand the body properly, we may find, by means of iridology, that we are suffering from autointoxication and are in the greatest need of foods containing chlorine, sodium, potassium, magnesium, and fluorine. Those people who have a heavy bone structure should eat foods that are rich in sodium to prevent too much calcium from being assimilated.

The body has many ways of communicating with us. The skin can reveal symptoms such as feverish conditions in various areas of the body. The tongue and breath reveal disturbances. The saliva can be tested; the hair can be analyzed. All of these are signals from the body that show one or more needs, and there are other means of communication besides these.

LEARNING WHAT PEOPLE ARE LIKE

Not only do symptoms tell what is going on in a person's life. The physical characteristics of a person's body and face provide useful information.

Personology is the study of the personality characteristics that correspond to certain physical and facial features. It was founded in 1941 by Edward V. Jones of Los Angeles, who was a California judge and attorney. The idea of personology is to know how to get along with people.

The eyes, for example, are exceptionally revealing. When a person's eyes are deep set, that person is usually very serious-minded. People with large eyes rely primarily on feelings more than reason or logic. (You don't need to spank a child with large eyes if you motivate him with the right feelings.) When the outer corners of the eyes are pulled down, that indicates a critical person. Almond eyes show gentleness and sensitivity. If the upper eyelid folds double over itself, the person tends toward being analytical.

The eyes of friendly people are often low, while the "highbrow" (actually, high eyebrow) has few friends and is hard to get acquainted with. A rounded eyebrow shows that a person has dramatic ability. A level, steady gaze indicates a person of sincerity and great energy, one who believes in himself.

Tactfulness is more common in a person with a narrow forehead. People with round foreheads like other people and make friends easily. People who prefer things generally have flat foreheads.

Tight-lipped people don't talk much, and a person with a big, square jaw is generally friendly and open, and primarily interested in the physical side of life. People with large lips like to talk, while those with "knob ends" on their noses are nosy. Self-reliance is shown by people who have flaring nostrils, and they are reliable. They are so dedicated that they will overwork and deplete their physical resources if they aren't careful!

Knowing such things about people makes it easier to understand what they may have done to contribute to their own health problems. It also helps us know how to communicate better with them and how to help them overcome health problems.

Just as spontaneous emotions are revealed by relatively quick changes in an individual's face and body posture, I believe more permanent characteristics are revealed by the unchanging structure of the face and body. These features, too, are forms of communication by our bodies, and they can exercise considerable influence on our health.

GETTING ALONG WITH PEOPLE

Each of us gets along better with some types of persons than others. It is important to see what these affinities are. There are certain affinities that must be taken into account to get along with a person, inside or outside of marriage. We should choose people who are good for us. There are some people whose behavior will drain you. You get sick when these people are around all the time. It is necessary that we associate with people who make us feel comfortable and with whom we are compatible. We need people who can keep us from fretting and worrying, people who feed us mentally as we journey through life. I believe that 50 percent of the people who come to me have negative feelings and hostilities for others around them. They could be in much better health and get really well if they could rid themselves of these feelings.

In speaking of these various people and how they act, we find there are some people who keep other people in suspense. They never express love, but appear self-sufficient, and even if grief is draining their vital forces, they tell no one. They put up a defensive act and may leave quickly without saying anything when offended. Such persons become gloomy in hot, humid, cloudy weather, but when it is dry and sunny, they are more affable. They are particular in dress and appearance, almost always have anxious moods, and are silently jealous. They keep their experiences to themselves, standing unrevealed to the world except for a few special friends. They are defensive—not offensive. Their systems are protective.

There are many things that we can see in people if we look at their type and mental attitude. There is a lot to learn, but it is an opportunity for us to observe how to read and understand the various ways in which the body communicates with us. We have given you a few ideas and tried to include those that most doctors need to understand a patient better.

The doctor himself has to be a person who communicates confidence, compassion, and empathy. He should be as healthy as possible and should be an influence to his patient by his example.

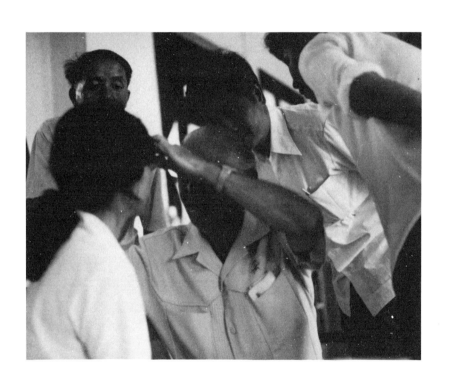

CHAPTER 14
Caring for Neglected Skin

Medical researchers are finally realizing how important the skin is, not only as a protective barrier to germs and other microorganisms, but as an eliminative channel, along with the bowel, kidneys, and lungs and bronchials. The skin is not only the largest organ of the human body; it is the one in which great numbers of nerve ends are found. For this reason, the skin gives symptoms of many different kinds whenever we have internal problems in the body.

The skin has other functions beside protecting the body from microorganisms and elimination of liquid wastes. It helps control body temperature through perspiration (cooling) and "goose bumps" (conserving heat). It helps regulate the liquid balance of the body, senses heat or cold in the environment (temperature), and helps people communicate with one another.

The skin can show what changes are going on inside the body. Liver spots or a bile rash appear on the skin. Severe gallbladder or liver problems can change the skin color to a yellowish tone. Dry, flaky skin, oily skin, boils, carbuncles, pimples, rashes, roughness, and scaly skin conditions are all common skin disorders.

PROBLEMS CAUSED BY THE THYROID

Thyroid disorders can cause skin problems. The skin can become dry, lacking the moisture content it should have. Many times the acupuncturist can take care of this problem. Of course, the iridologist must also make sure his patients are getting iodine-rich foods to assist in taking care of the thyroid. When the thyroid is taken care of, the skin is restored to its natural softness and pliability.

Many people don't realize how many problems can result from an underactive metabolism due to an iodine-deficient thyroid. When this condition persists, the normal skin moisturizing activity breaks down. There may be a gas problem in the body that is aggravating the dry skin condition.

Chronic problems with dry skin are the reason so many women have turned to moisturizing cosmetics, especially moisturizing creams. These can cause additional problems if unnatural chemicals are introduced into the skin.

THE SKIN IS THE "THIRD KIDNEY"

Many people don't realize how important the skin is in its eliminative function. Doctors sometimes call the skin our "third kidney." This eliminative function is most evident in cold weather when we notice that as we perspire less, we urinate more. When we perspire, we throw off a good deal of toxic material. When we don't perspire enough, the toxic material is forced into the tissues beneath the skin.

Researchers at major universities have recently "rediscovered" the skin, especially its eliminative function. They recognize that the skin is the single largest organ in the body, and they have found that perspiration is comparable to the elimination of the bowels and of the kidneys. Skin also contains the endings of many nerves and is easily irritated by chemicals, suntan lotions, cosmetics, ointments, and other unnatural substances.

The importance of skin elimination was highlighted in my own experience when a friend of mine was hospitalized with severe burns over half of his body. He died, but not of direct injury from the burns. The cause of his death was blood poisoning, uremia caused by the inability of the skin to eliminate.

Some years ago, an eight-year-old girl was completely covered with silver paint. She died of uremia. Her skin could not "breathe," or eliminate.

During a recent trip to the People's Republic of China, I lectured at a hospital in Canton. There, I was informed that in traditional Chinese medicine, the skin is considered the main point of entry for disease. This, among other reasons, helps explain why acupuncture, the stimulation of key nerve centers by inserting needles into the skin, is considered so important in the Chinese health tradition. In recent years, acupuncture has become more integrated with modern therapies. It has been successfully used as an anesthetic in several million operations, with no undesirable side effects. The purpose of acupuncture and the healing rationale behind it is its efficacy in balancing energy systems in the body.

THE SCURF RIM

The relationship between the skin and the kidneys is familiar to the iridologist in his study of the scurf rim, which is the dark ring around the outside edge of the iris. The scurf rim indicates skin toxicity and is a sign that the skin is not eliminating as well as it should. I have never examined a patient who did not have a scurf rim.

I once had the privilege of examining the eyes of sixteen Catholic nuns, all on the same day. They had the darkest scurf rims I had ever seen! It occurred to me that this was caused by the black habits they were required to wear. Only the oval of their faces was exposed to the sun, air, and wind. Many of these ladies had been nuns for as long as sixty years, and the toxic encumbrance was very heavy in the skin.

SKIN PROBLEMS ARE ABUNDANT

Acne is common in this country, and so is psoriasis. Patients come to me with boils, pimples, and rashes. There are cortisone salves that will keep the skin from eliminating by driving the toxic materials back into the tissue again. I believe the skin moisturizers so popular today are possibly the basis for many of our skin disturbances.

When sunlight plays on the skin of people who have used too many drugs, skin reactions, moles, warts, and even low-grade skin cancer can result. If you read some suntan lotion labels, you will see that they contain mineral oil. In the past, mineral oil was directly considered as a cause for rectal cancer. However, many products still contain this oil. I believe it is the chemical reaction between the ultraviolet in sunlight and our oil-and-lotion-soaked skin that is causing so many of our troubles.

When I was in Hawaii, I saw thousands of people going to the beach every day, smothering themselves with scented mineral oil compounds, then soaking up the rays of the sun all day. I don't believe it is good to cook all day in the sun. At one time, the Hawaiians never used suntain oil. Skin cancers are a relatively recent problem for them.

THE BATTLE AGAINST CELLULITE

Cellulite is the name given to the deposits of fat in women's thighs and buttocks that result in a skin-dimpling effect. Some in the health arts claim that cellulite is a highly specialized form of fat caused by mineral deficiencies and toxic settlements in fatty tissue. Others say it is just plain fat. In any case, therapies promising to remove cellulite are multiplying rapidly these days, and a lot of money is being spent on them.

What Do We Know About Cellulite?

Dr. Neil Solomon, former secretary of Maryland's Department of Health and Mental Hygiene, extracted fat samples from 100 people, some from people with cellulite layers and some from people without cellulite. Laboratory analysis showed no difference between the cellulite samples and "normal" fat.

Creams, lotions, herbs, vitamins, and mineral supplements have so far not been shown to be effective in removing or reducing cellulite. Authorities in weight reduction say that no equipment, exercise, or treatment can reduce fat from one part of the body.

Diet, together with exercise, seems to be the safest, healthiest, and most effective way of removing or reducing cellulite. Always consult your doctor before starting such a program.

I believe the main problem with underactive skin and toxic buildup in the tissues beneath it (including fatty tissue) is caused by an underactive bowel, together with poor food habits, inadequate exercise, and poor circulation to the skin. Skin underactivity and subcutaneous toxic deposits may be present whether or not cellulite is present. Cellulite is not caused by toxic deposits in tissue under the skin.

THE EFFECTS OF DRUGS AND PSORA ON THE SKIN

Skin problems are especially common among people who have taken many drugs internally. As drug residues work out through the skin, the sunlight reacts with these residues. There is a possible relationship between skin cancer and the taking of drugs, complicated by the inherited psoric taints from drugs that have been taken down through the generations.

The psora carried in the body, genetically inherited, sometimes settle in the skin. These may lead to further toxic accumulations. If we do not look to the causes of these troubles, I am convinced that they develop into skin cancers, psoriasis, and other chronic skin problems.

THE SKIN ABSORBS CHEMICALS

Several experiments have been done that prove that chemicals are absorbed through the skin.

Most of us know that garlic or onions eaten in a salad stay on a person's breath for hours, and the odor is often too strong for the comfort of others in the vicinity. Many years ago, when I was in Germany, I knew a man who experimented with raw garlic. He put it in his shoe, and put his foot back in the shoe. In a few minutes, the garlic could be detected on his breath, even though he hadn't eaten a bit of it. It had been absorbed through the skin.

At the Battle Creek Sanitarium, tests were done showing that chemicals could be absorbed through the skin and into the bloodstream. People put their feet in baking soda water for thirty seconds. Immediately after removing their feet from the water, they were given a urine test. The tests showed that bicarbonate of soda was in the urine.

Also at Battle Creek, turpentine packs were used on the back of a woman with kidney trouble. Thirty seconds later, turpentine showed up in her urine.

For years, many scientists thought that only water could be absorbed by the skin. That is not what tests have shown. Many experiments and tests have shown that skin does absorb substances other than water.

OUR SKIN IS OFTEN SUFFOCATED

We do not take care of our skin today. We suffocate it in nylon clothing. We pressurize it in belts and girdles. Fresh air is kept from the skin by the kinds of clothes we wear. We jump out of bed in the morning and put clothes on right away. When we go to bed at night, we put pajamas on. We don't usually give our bodies the exposure to the air and light necessary to have an active skin.

Women today are wearing nylon bras, and I am convinced that one consequence of these bras includes breast cancer, lumps, and cysts. I do not advise using nylon. Cotton bras would allow the skin to breathe.

Women who wear nylon panties and nylon pantyhose have had serious vaginal infections. Because of this, most manufacturers now include a cotton crotch in panties to improve air circulation.

I'm convinced that nylon hose are responsible for a lot of leg circulation problems. I'm also positive that cellulitis is often a result of wearing nylon clothing. Nylon clothing does not absorb sweat or allow the elimination that should take place through the skin.

The skin is not usually considered in our understanding of health and disease. Maybe we have come to think that our problems are all on the inside of the body. We need to look again.

WHAT DO BODY ODORS INDICATE?

Powerful chemicals are used to curtail underarm odors. These chemicals not only prevent odors, but prevent needed toxic elimination as well. If body odor is really bad, this may indicate a problem with underactivity in our other elimination channels. Bowel constipation is often found along with serious body odor.

Many people are also concerned about foot odor. In the soles of the feet and the palms of the hands are the largest pores in the entire body. The hands are exposed to air, but the feet are enclosed all day. When elimination through the bowel, kidneys, and bronchials is poor, foot odor will be worst.

UNUSUAL SKIN TREATMENTS

About forty years ago in Germany, I witnessed a skin treatment in which twenty-five gold needles attached to a spring were released to puncture the skin over a place where toxic material was believed to be stored. The punctures were only about one-eighth of an inch deep, and oil was immediately put on the punctures. In a day or two, a huge boil would develop and come to a head, increasing the speed of toxic elimination. This procedure was used on the face, the back, and other parts of the body.

While traveling in China, not long ago, I saw a similar method. The Chinese put a heated stick inside a glass or copper cup, and the cup was quickly pressed onto the skin. As the air cooled inside this glass or cup, a strong vacuum would develop, and the suction of this vacuum on the skin would draw the toxic material up to a head and through the skin. This was done on various parts of the body. The process is called moxibustion.

The idea of skin care differs in Eastern and Western medicine. When we in the West have a skin problem, we put something on it. We usually try to relieve the itching, stop the irritation, and reduce the swelling. This type of care may be considered a remedy without a correction, which always invites more problems. We should be taking care of the conditions inside us that relate to the skin problem.

The scurf rim, seen in an examination of the iris, is probably the clearest evidence we have of toxic material settling in and under the skin. I am convinced that this condition is so common because of the use of clothing. I do not mean that we should go without clothing and join a nudist camp, but there are good methods of taking care of the skin, such as skin brushing.

SKIN BRUSHING

No one can really have skin that is as healthy as it should be in today's civilization. Exposure to toxic air and washing with the toxic soaps and chemicalized water found today damage our skin. The pores are clogged by soaps and lotions, and elimination is hindered. So, we need to have a way to cleanse the skin without leaving it more toxic than we found it. This is best done by skin brushing.

Go to the natural food store and buy a long-handled vegetable bristle brush. Never use a nylon-bristle brush for skin brushing.

Start by brushing the hands, feet, and legs vigorously. Notice how alive the skin feels as you brush it. Notice the tingling feeling! Next, brush your torso, back, sides, and front. Ladies, avoid the breasts in brushing. Gentlemen and ladies, avoid both the genital area and the face. (You may wish to buy a soft-bristled brush for the face.) Brush for about five minutes before showering or taking a bath in the morning.

Brushing the skin removes the uric acid crystals, catarrh, and other acid wastes that come up through the pores of the skin. I recommend this as "dry bathing." You can do it twice a day, if you desire.

We build new skin every day, and brushing the skin twice daily helps the body to eliminate, get rid of old skin cells, and keep pores open. Some patients told me they had begun to perspire again after skin brushing, when they hadn't been perspiring for years.

INHERENTLY WEAK SKIN

Along with the rest of the body, the skin is subject to inherent weakness. Every person who comes to me as a patient has a scurf rim, which shows that the skin is in various levels of underactivity.

The skin is underactive because of mineral depletion and retention of metabolic toxins. The retardation of elimination causes further buildup of septic matter in and beneath the skin, which, in turn, causes further underactivity.

Unless something is done to reverse this condition, the skin continues its downward journey, growing worse and worse until symptoms appear—dryness, rash, scales, or worse. The skin, like other eliminative organs, has a "normal" transit time, a rate of throwing off perspiration that is comparable to the kidneys' rate of passing urine and the bowel's rate of elimination. When this transit time is impeded, a vicious cycle from increased underactivity to increased toxicity and increased deficiency takes place. Each makes the other worse. The eventual result is breakdown.

WHAT CAN WE DO TO HELP THE SKIN?

To take care of an underactive skin, several steps should be taken simultaneously. First, the efficiency of the bowel and kidneys can be increased by implementation of tissue cleansing methods and by proper feeding and exercise. Then, we should use a skin brush twice a day, as previously described.

Last, the skin must be fed to take care of its deficiencies, especially silicon deficiency. Silicon is the most important element in the skin.

Foods highest in silicon include alfalfa sprouts (and all other sprouts), whole grains, beans, rice bran, legumes, oat straw tea, figs, seeds, strawberries, and watermelon. The following foods also contain a measurable amount of silicon:

- Alfalfa tea
- Apples
- Apricots
- Asparagus
- Barley
- Beans
- Beets
- Beet greens
- Cabbage
- Cauliflower
- Celery
- Millet
- Oats
- Onions
- Parsnips
- Plums
- Raisins
- Psyllium seeds (ground)
- Pumpkin
- Pumpkin seeds
- Rice
- Rice bran

- Cherries
- Corn
- Cucumbers
- Dandelion greens
- Dates
- Figs
- Kelp
- Leaf lettuce

- Rice polishings
- Spinach
- Sunflower seeds
- Tomatoes
- Turnips
- Wheat bran
- Whole wheat

Remember, each organ in the body works with every other organ. If one organ is not healthy, the others will suffer. The skin is the largest organ, and one of the most important. It should not be neglected.

CHAPTER 15
The Brain and Nerves

The brain and nerves are the most highly-evolved tissues in the human body, designed to send and receive the electromagnetic vibrations that direct all the physiological functions of the body and allow man to creatively adapt to and alter his environment. It would take a building the size of a New York skyscraper to house a computer large enough to duplicate the brain's many functions. The human brain is truly a miracle of the evolutionary process.

V.G. Rocine considered the brain and its faculties central to his system of thought. The brain, he believed, is the physical vehicle through which the attributes of the soul are expressed and developed. Many famous philosophers, such as Plato and Descartes, held similar beliefs. Physical brain centers exist that are (or can be) awakened, nurtured, activated, and refined through training and experience so that the life of the soul can be given creative expression at the physical level. These same brain centers will remain as latent potentials if they are neglected.

Not only does Rocine's system of temperaments depend upon this view of the brain and its faculties, but his nutritional concepts are taken from it as well. Each organ and tissue structure of the body is connected via the nervous system to a specialized part of the brain that directs its function. Thus, we have a "heart brain," a "kidney brain," a "stomach brain," and so forth, and electromagnetic messages constantly pass back and forth along the autonomic nerves, telling the brain the state of each organ and tissue area. The brain responds by instructing the organ to adjust itself, not only in accordance with what is going on in that organ alone, but in consideration of the needs of all other organs and tissues in the body. Here, again, is another reason why we must take the wholistic approach in all healing. No single organ or tissue can be treated in isolation.

If the stomach lacks sodium, then we need to eat more sodium foods, but we must also consider the brain and nervous system as well. If the brain is anemic, or not being fed the right nutrients, the stomach center in the brain may not be operating properly. If the spine is out of alignment, the nerves may not be transmitting information properly from the stomach to the brain (or vice versa), and we may need chiropractic adjustment. Rocine was fully aware of the reflex activity between the brain and body structures, and his system takes that into account.

THE BRAIN AND INHERITANCE

Each person is born with a certain genetic endowment that determines the inherent strengths and weaknesses of the body and the overall constitutional strength. This is most clearly evident in iridology, the science of reading tissue structure and condition from the iris. The eye is an extension of the brain. We can tell by the arrangement of fibers in the iris which organs and tissues are inherently strong or weak. The brain itself is also a product of inheritance, and certain of its features may be inherently weak or strong, which will have an effect on various organs and systems in the body. The sum total of constitutional strength and inherent strengths and weaknesses determines our overall health potential and, to some extent, our temperament, which is also influenced by our family, friends, and education.

We must not make the mistake of assuming that inherent weaknesses, or a modest level of constitutional strength, are handicaps. Rather, they are opportunities. Each of us is gifted with enough talents and abilities to carry out the work our soul needs to express in this life. If a person has a weak stomach and digestive system, wisdom dictates that he should learn to take proper care of it and get on with the business of life. Our inherent strengths take care of themselves, and we must take care of our inherent weaknesses in order to overcome or compensate for them. We can do what we were meant to do in this life with what we have been given.

We can't take a strict physiological view of the brain without including some of its essential needs and qualities. Yes, the brain needs certain chemical elements and nutrients to function properly, but it also needs beauty, color, love, and companionship. We can't get all of the good out of our food unless we feel good about ourselves and our lives. To feel good, we must express the soul qualities and brain potentials we have inherited. If a silicon person is having skin problems, I can tell him to take more of the silicon foods, but I may also need to tell him he should go out dancing more often. Silicon people love to dance, and when you take that away from them, they can become frustrated, depressed, morose, and bored. I believe we live on what goes forth from us, and all of us have inherited the need to express ourselves in certain ways through our work, hobbies, play, and social relationships. We inherit these needs to express, just as we inherit our anatomy and physiology. To thwart an inherited gift or ability is to risk the kind of frustrated despondency that hinders relationships and invites disease.

The study of Personology is helpful when trying to find out more about people and their aptitudes. Personology analyzes the soul's influence on the development of the physical body. It was founded in 1941 by Edward V. Jones, a California judge and attorney from Los Angeles. I studied with Judge Jones for three years.

As a young attorney, Judge Jones began studying the relationship between physical character, personality, and behavior in 1909. He tried to discover what kinds of jobs people were best suited for. Over a period of thirty years he interviewed, analyzed, and tested nearly 10,000 people before making his findings public.

Judge Jones discovered that the eyes, nose, mouth, chin, ears, and forehead tell a great deal about our temperament and character. He based his studies on the reading of personality and character traits from the symmetry, size, location, and design of various parts of the face and body. Our looks, as well as our actions, likes, and dislikes, express our inherited qualities. More about Personology can be found in Chapter 13.

V.G. Rocine, my teacher, held the belief that all distinct temperament types were a result of chemical imbalance or chemical variance from the hypothetical "normal person" he took as his standard of comparison. To a considerable degree, this is inherited, impressed upon the structure of the brain and the DNA in each cell in the body.

I believe persons with constitutionally weak bodies or unique patterns of inherent weaknesses are fitted for specific occupations, marriages, and relationships. People are suited for certain climates, exercises, recreations, altitudes, and surroundings that will satisfy them, keep them healthy and happy, and allow the most productive use of their gifts. Inherent weaknesses serve to focus attention on one or more aspects of life that can become guiding principles in what we do, revealing the path we are to take in life. We must realize that inherent weaknesses are as valuable to us as inherent strengths in terms of their function as guideposts to the path of life most suited to us.

For example, I inherited a weak lung structure from my mother and, as a young man, I developed such serious lung problems that I was given up to die by doctors. It was my intense search for a healthy way to live that led me into the health work that has occupied my entire life since that time. After learning to overcome my own problems, my goal became to help others overcome theirs. An inherent weakness prompted me to take a path that has enabled me to help thousands of others.

In sum, the inherited qualities of our brains and temperaments determine the paths we can take in life, and the primary business of life is to discover the path that is uniquely right for each of us. Latent brain potentials can only be awakened by training and experience, but they offer great opportunity for soul growth.

ROCINE'S BRAIN CENTERS

V.G. Rocine taught that some brain centers must be developed to allow the proper expression of others. You may or may not believe in the existence of such centers, but I do. My sanitarium work at the Ranch, through which so many found their way back to health, was quite an operation, requiring about forty employees at one time. As a result, I had to develop *Precinoia*—the business center in my brain—to be able to help more people.

I learned about such brain centers from my teacher, V.G. Rocine, and have presented his list of centers. (See following list.) Rocine had simply assumed the division of the brain into functional centers which he grouped into logical subdivisions and named, using common classic Greek roots and prefixes, much in the same manner as medical science has named parts of the anatomy.

For example, *cardiophrenia*, the Heart Brain center listed under the Physical Group 1, is composed of the Greek-derived words, *cardio* (heart) and *phrenia* (brain). Cardiophrenia is an actual brain center located in the medulla oblongata of the brain, which controls the heart rate. In contrast, *Cheronia*, the joy center under Transcendental Group 6, must be considered a subjective subdivision of the "emotional brain" or limbic system, made up of the actual brain structures that curve around the corpus callosum, the wide band of tissue that connects the two hemispheres. *Cheronoia* is composed of the two Greek words *chero* (joy) and *noia* (mind), joined to create the technical term Rocine wanted. There may or may not be an actual "joy center" in the brain, but there is a section of the brain called the limbic system to which scientists attribute most if not all of our actual experienced emotions. The limbic system is made up of the *cingulate gyrus, the isthmus, the hippocampal gyrus, the uncas, and the hippocampus.* If this sounds like Greek to you, it is Greek. The classification of much of the terminology of anatomy—and disease—makes use of the Greek system of prefixes and roots.

Physical Group 1
- Cardiophrenia (Heart Brain Center)
- Pneumophrenia (Lung Brain Center)
- Tachiphrenia (Muscle Brain Center) speedbrain; motorium.
- Physical Senses (Perceptual Centers) the avenue of the soul in matter —touch, smell, hearing, taste, sight.
- Sensations (Sensory Center) kinesthesia, balance, other internal somatic senses.

Industrial Group 2
- Benoia (Health Center) the faculty that loves life and health.
- Alonoia (Trophic Center) the faculty of nutrition.
- Hygronoia (Hydric Center) the faculty that studies the watery creation.
- Precinoia (Business Center) the business faculty.
- Senoia (Intronoic Center).
- Warnoia (Safety Center) the faculty-voice of "safety first."
- Eceonoia (Home Center) the home and nationloving faculty.

Associative Group 3
- Besnoia (Sex Brain Center) the faculty that loves life and health.
- Philnoia (Love Center) the love, marriage and family faculty.
- Hebenoia (Parental Center) the motherhood and nursing faculty.
- Synnoia (Fraternal Center) the faculty of mind unification.

Volitive or Executive Group 4
- Leonoia (Power Center) the faculty of power, will and daring.
- Cacnoia (Bolic Center) the faculty that senses evil.
- Stonia (Stoic Center) the faculty of science and stability.
- Connoia (Connoic Center) the faculty of mind unity.

Exalative Group 5
- Autonoia (Autonoic Center) the faculty that leads and governs.
- Lausnoia (Fame Center) the faculty that craves fame and popularity.
- Uranoia (Scenic Center) the faculty that studies the universe.
- Kalosnoia (Beauty Center) the soul faculty that judges beauty.

Transcendental Group 6
- Elnoia (Adorative Center) the faculty of divine wisdom.
- Eldinoia (Eldic Center) the faculty that loves the past.
- Cheronoia (Joy Center) the soul faculty of joy and optimism.
- Eunoia (Service Center) the faculty of serving others.
- Telenoia (Psychic Center) the faculty of "second sight."
- Nomonoia (Law Center) the soul's law faculty.

Perceptive Group 7
- Spectomanas (Object Center) the faculty that notices objects.
- Rupamanas (Morphic Center) the faculty that remembers form and shape.
- Metromanas (Space Center) the faculty that judges size, room and space.
- Kinemanas (Motion Center) the faculty that studies force and motion.

- Taximanas (System Center) the order and system faculty.
- Plurimanas (Account Center) the soul's accountant faculty.
- Lokamanas (Place Center) the soul's geographer and map.
- Chromanas (Color Center) the color perceiving faculty.
- Theromanas (Heat Center) the faculty that senses heat.

Expressive Group 8
- Phonomanas (Sound Center) the soul's faculty for sound.
- Kalamanas (Time Center) the time faculty; the soul's chronologist.
- Logomanas (Speech Center) the faculty of speech; word memory.
- Phenomanas (Phenic Center) the faculty that notices what happens.

Philomatic Group 9
- Theamanas (Mimic Center) relating to God in man.
- Tuimanas (Physiognostic Center) the soul's physiognomist (a faculty).
- Suamanas (Suave Center) the faculty of courtesy and good manners.
- Lilamanas (Wit Center) the faculty of wit; sense of contrasts.
- Tectomanas (Building Center) the faculty of constructive reason.
- Lipimanas (Analytic Center) the faculty of analysis and induction.
- Hetumanas (Causation Center) the faculty of causation.

Obviously, it can be argued that some of these brain centers of Rocine's construction do not exist. Also, *Hetumanas,* the "causation center," may be far more complex than a single center in the brain could account for. Brain researchers have been unable to pin down any part of the human brain that can be said to initiate a thought, idea, or action.

Regardless of what you think of Rocine's system of brain centers and categories, he was using state-of-the-art knowledge of brain anatomy and physiology in his time, and many of his categories make logical sense if not physiological sense. Time marches on and knowledge changes, but these categories have helped me understand how the brain/mind is affected by inherent weaknesses, chemical deficiencies, and toxic settlements. Consequently, I have developed my own system of brain/mind categories of centers, each with its own set of qualities.

EXTENDING THE WORK OF ROCINE

In my own work in iridology, one of the greatest challenges has been to elaborate upon the brain area that extends from eleven to one o'clock in my iris chart (Figure 3.1). The brain area of the iris is the area that is least understood and developed. Using Rocine's idea of brain centers as a "seed" concept, I developed a system of brain flairs to demonstrate both the high-level (beneficial) and low-level (non-beneficial) expressions of the faculties I believe are found in and expressed through the brain.

The dictionary gives one definition of "flair" as "a natural talent or aptitude; bent; knack" and another definition as "an instinctive discernment." I consider the main category or brain center as "the flair." The qualities characteristic of each brain flair are simply forms of its expression.

In my system, each brain flair is identified with a particular area of my iris chart between eleven and one o'clock, which in turn is identified with an actual portion of brain anatomy, together with its known physiological functions. This is not very thoroughly worked out in iridology at this point in time, but I believe it will be. I am leaving this task for someone else to do in the future.

My concept of brain flairs has been described more completely in my book *Iridology: The Science and Practice in the Healing Arts, Volume II.* One category is presented in Table 15.1. The category is called the Animation and Life Center (or Vitality Center).

Table 15.1   Animation and Life (Vitality Center)

Low Level Expression	High Level Expression
Gloom	Ecstacy
Complaining	Joy
Depression	Love
Fatigue	Vitality
Enervation	Physical energy
Forgetfulness	Mental energy
Despondency	Enjoyment
Listlessness	Nerve/gland center
Hopelessness	Liveliness
Pessimism	Cheerfulness
Fearfulness	Optimism
Fussiness	Spiritual center
Indifference	Unity center for body,
Unsociability	mind, spirit
Stupor	Enthusiasm
Heaviness in head	Memory
Melancholy	
Sadness	
Morbidity	
Apprehension	
Discouragement	
Disgust	

Other brain flairs shown in my iris chart are Sensory/Locomotion, Inherent Mental, Equilibrium/Dizziness Center, Sex Impulse/Mental Sex, Five-Sense Area, Ego Pressure, Acquired Mental/Speech, Mental Ability and Medulla.

The Animation and Life Center (or Vitality Center) at twelve o'clock in the irides, is the great "general barometer" of health, representing a cluster of the most important brain structures and functions. The part of the sensory-motor cortex serving the leg, knee, and foot; the limbic system or "emotional brain"; the corpus callosum, which connects the brain hemispheres; and parts of the thalamus, hypothalamus, pituitary gland, midbrain, and pons are located here. Because of anemia, poor nutrition, tumor, disease, or nerve problems, this area of the brain is the first to be affected, and when its functioning is depressed, the symptoms of low-level expression in the preceding list are evident.

Fatigue is the first and most obvious symptom. All sick people are fatigued. When we realize that the pleasure center, the appetite center, and the endocrine system control center are all found in this part of the brain (the Vitality Center), we realize that any disturbance of this center is very serious and must be taken care of.

The faculties listed in my brain flair work are intended to help show which brain centers are involved in particular health problems and conditions. As the causes are corrected through diet, exercise, mechanical treatments, rest, and other measures, we can begin to look for the higher level expressions to appear, indicating progress. When the healing arts understand how to interpret symptoms of brain/mind dysfunction and take care of them, we will see a great new day in terms of effective results in healing. Like V.G. Rocine, I am convinced that taking care of the brain is the key to rejuvenating the body.

ALZHEIMER'S DISEASE

Alzheimer's disease, also called presenile dementia, afflicts about 1.5 million people in the United States, 5 percent of the population over age sixty-five and 60,000 younger victims. The youngest known case is twenty-eight years old. Early symptoms are forgetfulness and mood changes, while later on, almost complete loss of memory and other brain functions takes place. Stress or depression speeds up the onset of this condition, and Western medicine regards it as incurable and irreversible. Once it starts, the disease takes from a few months to four or five years to bring a person to complete helplessness.

Although the cause of the disease is so far unknown, autopsies show an accumulation of abnormal fibers in some nerve cells of the brain's cerebral cortex, scattered degeneration of nerve endings, a shortage of choline acetyltransferase (which affects memory), and an excess of aluminum.

One study showed six times the normal amount of aluminum deposited in the brains of those with Alzheimer's disease. This condition afflicts men, women, the rich, the poor, and all races equally. Some researchers believe it may involve a chromosomal defect.

Possible Causal Factors

The brain is affected by many factors, including heredity, food, exercise, overwork, fatigue, and gravity. Because Alzheimer's disease has been only recently identified, we can't say whether or not cases of the disease have increased in the past century. It may have been identified previously as mental disease or senility, so we can't say it is caused by some particularly modern phenomenon such as processed foods, except in the sense that processed foods lower everyone's resistance to disease.

Alzheimer's disease is possibly linked to arteriosclerosis, the buildup of fatty deposits on the walls of arteries, which blocks small blood vessels completely and cuts off nutrient supplies from cell groups in peripheral tissue. Lecithin, a phospholipid that contains choline, can dissolve the fatty deposits, but it is destroyed in foods by processing or heating. Another component of the problem, I believe, is anemia and poor circulation, which keeps the brain from getting all the oxygen and nutrients it needs. An overworked, overtired brain in someone who has a desk job is likely to be accompanied by lack of adequate circulation and oxygenation of the blood due to insufficient exercise. Add heavy smoking, drinking of alcoholic beverages, and consumption of heavy, high-fat, meat-and-starch meals late in the afternoon or evening, and you have a prime candidate for Alzheimer's disease. We could add heavy use of salt and the drinking of four to eight cups of coffee a day to the lifestyle just described.

Iridology has shown in such cases a heavy sodium/cholesterol ring in the brain area, accompanied by the bluish arcus senilis, indicating anemia. I do not believe these things are incurable, but I understand why drug therapy has, so far, not worked well. Drugs will not get to the affected part of the brain if the small blood vessels are plugged and circulation to the head is poor.

One study has shown that a healthy diet (excluding coffee, alcohol, refined carbohydrates, fatty meats, etc.), plus megadoses of vitamins and some mineral supplements, brought increased vigor, restored memory, and stimulated better mental function to five out of eight persons with Alzheimer's disease. I believe it is possible to extend this natural approach considerably farther for better benefits.

First, the bloodstream needs to be cleansed, and we do this by bowel cleansing, diet changes, and chelation therapy, if indicated. Second, we need to build up the blood with foods high in iron (to raise the red blood count and pick up more oxygen) and get it circulating with regular physical exercises, and slanting board exercises (to get the blood to the head area). Deep breathing exercises and use of the bouncer (mini-trampoline) would get more oxygen into the blood for burning up fatty deposits in blood vessels. We can also take extra lecithin and some high density fats to help dissolve fatty deposits.

These are not methods that will give quick, dramatic results in a week or two (except possibly chelation and bowel cleansing), but slow, steady progress should come with excellent results in a year's time. Nature is slow, but sure.

HOW THE BRAIN AND NERVES WORK

The human brain, about the size of a softball, weighs roughly two-and-three quarter pounds and contains ten billion neurons. The brain uses 20 percent of the body's blood, 25 percent of the oxygen, and is energized by glucose. If the blood supply, oxygen, or glucose is cut off, brain damage occurs in a matter of minutes.

The brain and nervous system work by means of electromagnetic signals that travel along nerve pathways to specific destinations, depending on the type of signal. Neurons, like other cells, have a cell body and nucleus, but unlike other cells, they have a single long "leg" called an axon and several shorter "legs" called dendrites. Signals go one way—they are picked up by dendrites and flow through the axon to the next neuron's nucleus or dendrites, jumping a gap called a synapse, in which a chemical medium is required to pass the signal along. Here, things get very interesting.

At the synapse, the axon releases a chemical (such as acetylcholine) into the gap until it contacts the membrane of the dendrite, altering its electrical potential. Sodium, outside the membrane, and potassium, inside the membrane, shift sides. Both are electrically charged, and the exchange of places polarizes the membrane and allows the electromagnetic nerve impulse to pass across the gap and into the next dendrite. After the signal goes by, another chemical named cholinesterase is released to break down the acetylcholine, so that the electrical potential of the membrane is restored and ready for the next signal. (The fastest nerve impulses travel about eighty miles per hour; slower nerves may only move at the rate of four miles per hour.)

All chemicals (there are several) that help signals cross synaptic gaps are called neurotransmitters; chemicals that stop signals from passing are called neuroinhibitors. Both are important in the brain and nervous system, and we must realize that the right chemical substances must be available for the nervous system to work right. Nerve conduction is chemical as well as electrical.

Excess acidity or alkalinity in the body can increase or decrease nerve excitability. Depression of the nervous system can result in coma, while overstimulation can lead to convulsions. Alcohol and caffeine cause an increase in the frequency of nerve impulse generation, while tranquilizers and various other hypnotic drugs reduce them.

Many nerves are surrounded with a fatty, myelin sheath, made largely of lecithin, that increases the speed of nerve transmission. The gray matter in the brain is made up of bare nerve bodies and axons, while the white matter is myelinated fibers, insulated fibers, like the insulation around electrical wires. In the gray matter, the uninsulated nerve fibers interact with each other electromagnetically, influencing one another's vibrations, increasing some and diminishing others, cancelling them out.

The brain contains centers for sight, sound, smell, taste, touch, and speech, plus others for balance, movement, and so forth. Thinking goes on in the cortex, mostly the frontal cortex, the outer thin layer that covers the cerebrum, which includes the two large hemispheres. Memory is distributed broadly throughout the brain. The emotional center is the limbic system, surrounding the part of the brain that connects the two hemispheres. Jutting up from the end of the spinal column into the midbrain is a section of brain called the reticular formation, which has to do with the wake/sleep system, alertness, and primitive functions such as fight or flight. The cerebellum, at the lower posterior of the brain, has to do with crude muscle coordination; together with the cerebrum, it works to tune and control muscles to a high degree of coordination.

In the center of the brain, roughly "between the ears," we find a set of supremely important brain structures: thalamus, hypothalamus, pineal gland, and pituitary gland. The thalamus is a relay center for sensory information, and crude recognition of pain, temperature, and touch. The pineal gland in the thalamus is our biological clock and psychic center, tuning into visual impulses to generate production of certain hormones and biochemicals needed by the brain and body. The hypothalamus, under the thalamus, regulates the amount of water in the body, the temperature, appetite, electrolyte concentrations, and much of our emotional expression and behavior. It is in the hypothalamus that nerve impulses stimulate production of neurohormones of several types that activate the pituitary, the "master gland" of the endocrine system, to release its own hormones regulating other endocrine glands—such as the thyroid, parathyroids, islets of Langerhans in the pancreas, adrenals, ovaries, and testes. So the hypothalamus, we find, exerts a great deal of control over sexuality and metabolism through interaction with the pituitary.

Together, the thalamus, hypothalamus, pineal, and pituitary acts as a "grand central station" in the brain, receiving information from all body organs, tissues, and systems; all sensory organs; and the memory, association, and thinking portions of the brain. (It is due to the thalamus and hypothalamus that nerves to the iris are able to reflexly represent the condition of all body organs, glands, and structures.) These same brain structures, correlating all this information, largely regulate all autonomic functions—the automatic functions of heart, lungs, liver, pancreas, spleen, and so forth—as well as much of our conscious behavior. It is in the hypothalamus that our thoughts, emotions, autonomic functions, perceptions, memories, and behavior integrate into what we call consciousness or soul expression, and this is also the psychosomatic center where thoughts influence every cell of the body.

We are not trying here to give a total picture of the brain and its functions, but a sort of overview. The brain is the most important organ in the body. The medulla, or chest brain, contains a heart center, lung center, vasoconstriction center, and many reflex activity centers such as those of coughing, sneezing, and vomiting. It also connects to the thalamus and cerebellum, which influence its functions and which are, in turn, influenced by it.

All the brain centers that Rocine found, all the faculties that I have elaborated on, as well as the emotional, behavioral, somatic, and psychosomatic centers and functions of the brain are affected by five main things. They are: what the spirit knows to be true, what the soul needs to express, what the body experiences in its environment, what the state of health is, and what nutrients are being brought in.

Speaking strictly of the physical level, the brain, mind, soul, and spirit can do nothing unless the brain is fed properly. Speaking strictly of the spiritual and mental levels, the right foods will do the brain little good unless we are on a path leading to truth, love, joy, peace, and service to mankind. The spiritual, mental, and physical aspects cannot be separated. We must think wholistically.

FEEDING THE BRAIN

As the highest-evolved tissue in the body, the brain needs the highest-evolved foods. The calcium and phosphorus that build the bones cannot build good brain structure and function. The bones can do well on calcium and phosphorus from plant life, but the brain needs the biochemicals derived from animal life. It is possible that we can get some good out of nuts and seeds in the brain, but it can only happen when the enzymes are activated, and the vibratory rate has been raised.

The brain is basically a phosphorus organ, and phosphorus is the great "light bearer." The brain needs light, speed, and electromagnetism. The best brain foods are fish (especially from the sea, with white meat, fins, and scales), codfish roe, egg (especially the yolk), goat milk, cheese (the kind that crumbles), and lean meat.

In addition to phosphorus, the brain needs the nerve fats such as cholesterol and lecithin, which balance each other out. Cholesterol is needed in the formation of hormones such as cortisol and progesterone, as well as in the white matter of the brain. Cholesterol is a lipid sterol, whereas lecithin is a phospholipid, containing phosphorus and choline. Lecithin is needed to keep cholesterol in a semi-liquid state, or it can harden, as it tends to do on the walls of arteries in arteriosclerosis.

The choline in lecithin is needed in the brain to produce acetylcholine, the neurotransmitter we have previously discussed. Researchers have found lecithin to be helpful in treating Alzheimer's disease in roughly 30 percent of the cases, and in treating Parkinson's disease. The brain also needs high-quality proteins—amino acids and RNA—as energy resources. White sugar, alcohol, and caffeine overstimulate the brain temporarily, then leave it drained and underactive. They function more as toxins than foods.

The nerves and brain need calcium to maintain the permeability of the cells. That is, calcium is needed before cells can take in the proper amounts of other nutrients and release metabolic wastes. Calcium often works together with phosphorus, which acts as an energy-transfer catalyst in the metabolism of starches and proteins. Calcium keeps us grounded and motivated for success. We can't keep up our courage and determination without calcium, which gives us the determination to carry things through. Phosphorus helps us think; calcium helps us translate the thought into successful action.

Sodium and potassium are essential to the proper functioning of nerves at the synapse junctions, where they diffuse in and out of cell membranes to help nerve signals pass. We must obtain these from foods, not table salt, salt substitutes, or inorganic tablets. Okra, whey, celery, and goat's milk are good sources of organic sodium and potassium, and bananas are a good source of potassium.

We need manganese in the brain for two reasons. First, it is the love element. In experiments, manganese-deficient rats refused to nurse their young, allowing them to die or even killing them. Manganese helps develop the parental center of the brain. It is also necessary for a good memory. Manganese is found in nuts and seeds, especially Missouri black walnuts. It is also found in seafood.

The nerves and brain are electromagnetic in function, and require silicon. The outsides of the nerves use silicon, called "the magnetic element," to increase effective nerve conduction. Sprouts, seeds, nuts, and the other husks of grains have a good deal of silicon, especially rice polishings. We must have enough silicon for the brain and nerves to have that magnetism we need in our relationships with others.

We need sulphur foods—eggs, cauliflower, leeks, garlic, and onions—to build up the "go" of the brain. When the medulla begins to break down, one of the first things we find is a changeable pulse, skipping heartbeats, and uneven breathing. One of the nicest remedies is coconut and nutmeg, and we can take sage tea and watermelon seed tea. We could also have some easily digested fish. If the sex center is breaking down, we need the sulphur foods, but we also need iron—parsley tea and black cherry juice are good. One of the very best brain and nerve tonics is an egg yolk in black cherry juice. This contains the iron, sulphur, cholesterol, and lecithin all at once, a wonderful combination. Asparagus and strawberries are also good.

RNA (ribonucleic acid) is reported to promote longevity and brain alertness, and its primary function in the cells is to build the proteins needed in cellular rejuvenation. Foods high in RNA include yeast, sardines, and microalgae such as spirulina and chlorella. Sardines feed on RNA-rich microorganisms from the sea and are high in protein, iodine, and a broad array of trace elements.

Once I visited Charlie Smith in Florida, who was 138 years old at the time. I asked, "Charlie, what is it that has given you your long life?" He answered, "The will of God has a lot to do with it, and I love the Lord. Besides that, I've lived on nothing but sardines and crackers for the past thirty years." It almost blew my mind to think of a person living for thirty years straight on sardines and crackers, but I believe he did it.

The importance of amino acids to the brain can be indicated by an example. Tryptophan, an essential amino acid, is important in producing natural sleep and in keeping depression away. When we take tryptophan, some of it is converted in the brain to the neurotransmitter serotonin, a vasoconstrictor which is active in the sleep-wake cycle. When the chemicals that help produce natural sleep are out of balance, insomnia and depression can result. This is counteracted by the natural effects of tryptophan, which promotes a natural sleep cycle, unlike the tranquilizers and sleeping pills that simply knock people out.

It has been suggested that tranquilizers, sleeping pills, and other relaxant drugs shield the brain from the stresses of everyday life, therefore contributing to the withdrawal of the mind from any involvement with any of the problems of normal existence. Besides reducing the brain's ability to cope with ordinary events of life, tranquilizing drugs may leave residues in the blood that can be transmitted through the mother to the offspring, laying the ground for potential drug addiction later, when the child grows up. Magnesium and phosphorus are two elements that are most important, along with the other elements, to the proper nourishment of the brain. They enable the brain to withstand the stresses and pressures of modern life. In other words, when we eat properly, we will not be bothered with nerve problems, fears, anxieties, and insomnia.

Feeding the brain and nerves is vitally important because the brain is the symphony conductor that leads the body. We cannot have a healthy body without a well-fed brain.

TREATING PATIENTS WITH MENTAL PROBLEMS

I have not had a lot of patients with mental problems in the past, but there have been some. I can tell you that those who have a good physical body and makeup, and have the best of health, are those with the fewest mental problems. Most of us tend to think that mental problems come from the mental and not the physical realm. However, we have to realize that we can't separate the mind and the body. Anyone who has a mental problem has to be taken care of from both a mental and physical standpoint. You can't resolve mental problems by only psychological therapy, because there are always corresponding physical problems such as nerve acids, glandular imbalances, mineral depletion, and toxicity problems to take care of before there is complete recovery. Resolving mental problems is not only a matter of taking care of the manic-depression, schizophrenia, nerve depletion, or other problem—it is a matter of getting the physical body straightened out and getting the path straightened out.

When we become depleted and starved for the chemical elements needed by our body, we soon find that our mental responses become abnormal. Some people are starving for "mental" things like kindness, acceptance, affection, love, beauty, and music. Any person can starve mentally as well as physically. It has been said, "Man does not live by bread alone," and that is true. We need mental nourishment as much as we need physical nourishment.

Also, some people need what I call replacement therapy—replacement of the old thoughts. They have to take up something new. In some cases, the rigid old patterns contribute to disease.

Case Number One

I'd like to review a few of my patients' cases and bring out some of the things we have to take care of. One lady, who was an aviatrix, came to us from the East. She had loved flying for many years, until her plane crashed. She survived the crash, but from then on she was not *wholly* alive. The crash put her in a state of shock, and she didn't pull out of it well. She decided she wasn't going to get in an airplane any more. She wouldn't even get into an automobile. She didn't want to travel at all.

When she came to my Ranch, I spent a lot of time building her up physically, because I feel that mental functions depend on brain functions, and the brain is a physical entity that has to be taken care of. It has to be fed.

As we began to take care of the mental depletion in this lady, I put her on a balanced food program, and she began showing a little improvement. After the second month, she was hiking through the hills around the Ranch. Her lung structure and circulation built up from the exercise, and her bowel activity was very good. Her blood test showed no sign of anemia, and she seemed to have reached a normal level of physical health.

Still, I wanted to see her start doing things such as traveling by auto. She finally consented to go for a ride, but that's as much as she wanted to do. When I asked her to drive the car, she refused. It was a matter of getting over a psychological hump. She had good physical health to work with, but how could we get past the obstacles or the mental blocks she created?

I drove about five miles with this lady one day. Then, I started to complain of a headache. I said it was impossible for me to continue driving, and I had to pull over. The lady was upset by the fact that she couldn't do anything for me. We were out on a road with no houses and no phones. She asked what she could do.

I told her there was only one thing to do, since I had to get back to the Ranch as soon as possible—she would have to drive me back. You wouldn't believe the fuss she put up at first! She said she couldn't drive. I said she just had to—it was an emergency. I showed her what had to be done and, of course, with her past mechanical knowledge, it was no trouble at all for her to get the car started and on our way. She drove me back to the Ranch.

In this situation, I sensed her sympathy and used it. Of course, this was an act on my part, but I went through with it to show her that she could drive. She had to be put in a situation where she had no choice but to do it. Her skill at driving was evident, even though she hadn't used it for a long time.

The next day, I told her, "Let's go down to the store. You drive." She took quite a delight in driving the car again! In another month, she had overcome all her fears, and another patient was sent home minus the problem she brought with her.

I recently read of a man who weighed over a thousand pounds. He has lost 400 pounds, but he doesn't want to stand up because he believes his legs will be too weak to hold his weight. The people trying to help him are being forced to try to get around his psychological blocks.

I have often seen these psychological blocks broken. But we can't do it well on just a fasting routine or a cleansing diet. Of course, we do need to detoxify the person, but mental problems require a high protein diet, which is exactly the opposite from an elimination diet. Building up the brain and nerves is very necessary in people with mental problems.

Some people have been carrying around mental blocks for years. The man who weighed over half a ton had been in this condition for the past twenty years, so he is bound to have developed some mental problems. It will be interesting to see how he changes as he gets used to a healthy, balanced diet. He can both lose weight and feel better about himself, I am sure, by using the proper foods and knowing each day that he is better and more capable. Everything must be taken step by step, and one step at a time. Finally, the man will have the confidence to go all the way.

The tissue must have sustenance. There is a time for elimination, a time for transition, and a time for building. There is a time for maintaining. We must see to our patients' needs, meeting them on the level where they exist.

Case Number Two

I had a patient once who was transferred from a mental institution. She was in a straitjacket because she was dangerous to herself and others, destructive in anything she did. Her mother was aware of my work and wanted to see whether an alternative approach would help her daughter. No progress was being made by keeping her in a straitjacket and drugged most of the time.

I knew about an unoccupied sanitarium, and I suggested to the mother that the girl be taken there. I said, "Let's rent it for a couple of months and get a couple of nurses to take care of her. Then, we can go through a daily routine, which will be good for her." We put her on a thirty-day fast, and her body went through a terrific cleansing. With the nutritional buildup and taking care of the brain and nerves, there was a wonderful nerve response and a wonderful change in her behavior.

At the end of the second month, the patient was able to walk and do things for herself. It was wonderful to see that she finally began to understand what we were doing, and started cooperating. She could tell she was progressing. One day, while I was walking with her, she asked me how she had gotten into this trouble.

I said, "If you were fixing a lunch for your husband, what would you put in his lunchbox?" She said, "I would put in sandwiches, a bottle of milk or a drink of some kind, and some fruit." I said, "Suppose that after you put this lunch together, and put it in his lunchbox, someone took the lunchbox and shook it up so everything inside was mixed up. When he opened it and saw what was there, what do you think he would say?"

She said, "He'd say, 'what a mess this is!'" I said, "Well, darling, that's what you were. You were a mess—a physical mess, a mental mess, and a spiritual mess, too. You came from a wonderful spiritual home, and there is no reason for you to have all of these problems. Now there's only one thing to do, and that's to get out of this mess. Let's find out what has to be done."

That was thirty years ago. I told her that one of the things she would have to do was make a decision about what to do with her husband, because he was largely responsible for the mess she had gotten into. Finally, the girl took it upon herself to divorce the man. She married again, a very wonderful man, and had children. Her life straightened out, and she had no return of her troubles since that time.

Case Number Three

A girl in Santa Monica had become mentally disturbed after having a baby. She was under the care of psychologists, and had to be housed and guarded because of her dangerous mental condition. When I was asked to take the case, I suggested that this girl's mother rent a home in a rural area south of Los Angeles so that we could take care of the girl from a physical standpoint.

We put her on a fast for twenty days, and she got rid of some tremendous problems during this period. She went through a number of little healing crises. After the eliminations, she began to get better and better. I could see that the care of the nurses had a good deal to do with it, because they made sure she had plenty of exercise, outdoor activities, and applications of cold and hot packs, working to build up a better circulation. I mention this because I feel that you cannot handle people with mental problems by reasoning with them. You cannot go in and tell them you are going to do this or that. Usually, their minds are not able to reason. You must start by working toward a clean body, and then the mind gradually begins to come back. And it works! That's why I keep using the elimination work, and believe in it.

At the end of thirty days, this girl went home. That was years ago, and she has not had any trouble since.

I could go through case after case and tell you wonderful things that happened, primarily as a result of balanced nutrition and exercise. When treating a patient with a mental disorder, we took care of the physical body first. By the fasting and elimination process, we got rid of many of the drugs that had settled in the body. These drugs had destructive effects upon the nerves and the brain, and tended to feed the problem and not help the patient. Drug-ridden people have such destructive minds that it takes an elimination to cleanse and clear drug residues out before they can get back to normal.

There isn't any person with mental problems who doesn't need physical care. Treating mental patients with drugs only gives them temporary relief and minimizes the amount of care they need from nurses. They can be put away in their room and no further care is required, but they don't get well. You have to work with these people to help them return to normal.

A VISIT TO RUSSIA

Once, I took an enlightening trip to Russia. While I was in Moscow, I was introduced to a Dr. Nicolaev by a good friend from Canada, Pete Maloff, who went along as my translator. In the doctor's office, Mr. Maloff introduce me as Dr. Jensen from the United States, a doctor who practiced iridology. Dr. Nicolaev said, "Really? You can't be the Dr. Jensen who wrote the books on cooking, foods, nutrition, and iridology, can you?" I said, "Yes." He threw his arms around me and said, "I never thought I'd have the opportunity to meet you. I want you to go with me and see what we are doing." We went to a mental institution, almost a block square and eight stories high, that Dr. Nicolaev was in charge of. He took us through one room after another.

There were about sixteen inmates in each room. Most were schizophrenic. As we came into the rooms, the people would all stand up at attention in their lemon-colored gowns. They told about their problems, and some talked about getting well and being able to leave the institution. Mr. Maloff translated what the patients said. They talked about how long they had been there and what treatment they were receiving.

We went through room after room, and Dr. Nicolaev told us how he had learned of my work by reading my books. When he began to apply my work in this institution, the healing rate increased greatly. He told me that 60 percent of the people in this institution had been able to leave and go back to their homes and jobs because of the dietetic care and nutrition work. I thought this was wonderful! We should try that in our country. It was nice to see that an alternative health care method, using some of my work, was used in a mental institution in Russia with good results. At the end of the tour, over 100 doctors came together, and I lectured to them on my work using nutrition as a basis for building a better integrity of all kinds of cell structure, whether in the respiratory system, the bowel, the brain, or nervous system.

I feel sorry for people who have become mentally disturbed and who become alcoholics or drug addicts. We find, to begin with, that we cannot get into the minds of these people easily. Reason is not the place to start, but reason returns if we work toward a clean body. We have to make sure they have the proper nerve supply and proper environment. We cannot live in this polluted world and expect a person with polluted tissues to react normally. He needs help in developing a new and better cell structure. He needs a cleaner environment to live in. We all do.

Many people today are being treated for manic depression. Many are on lithium and other mood-altering drugs. These people are only on a symptom-relief, case management program, with little hope for progress. We are not taking care of the basic problem in a way that brings a clean body and tissues that have the integrity to be normal.

THE NEUROGENETIC REFLEX

In my fifty-plus years as an iridologist, the area of the iris that represents the brain has fascinated and challenged me. The brain area of the iris is larger than the area of any other organ. I have wondered what the brain has to do with biochemical deficiencies in the body, and what it has to do with toxic settlements in inherently weak organs. I have given this a great deal of thought over the years.

There is conclusive evidence of a reflex activity involving the brain that actually *directs* toxins to be deposited in inherently weak organs when those parts of the body are lacking in biochemical elements. When we realize that nothing happens in the body unless the brain allows or directs it, we have to see the process as a reflex activity.

We must understand that in the original union of the sperm and ovum, the consequent development of the embryo proceeds in such a way that the brain develops at the same time that other organ tissue structures are being differentiated and formed. The "heart center" of the brain does not grow independently of the heart itself, and all other structures develop with the brain in this parallel but correlated manner. Inherent weakness in the body is correlated with inherent weakness in the brain in the corresponding center. We must also understand that inherently weak areas act as if their metabolism were slower—nutrients are not assimilated as well as in "normal" tissues and wastes are not eliminated as quickly. Similarly, weak brain areas are functionally depressed in their operation. They are not as efficient in directing the activities of the organs they supervise. So, the weakness is built in.

As long as toxic overload does not occur, the inherent weaknesses function with relative normalcy. But as soon as the body loads up with more catarrh, acid wastes, chemical toxins, and drugs than it can dispose of, the weakest channels of the body become routes for the deposition and storage of toxic wastes by the neurogenetic reflex. The nerves to a particular area reveal its inherent weakness or strength to the brain, and we can read this in his eyes, which are extensions to the brain.

The health of the mother plays a role in these processes. If the mother is chemically short in any element, this deficiency will affect the development of the embryo in the corresponding area. Keep in mind that each organ, tissue, and structure in the body has one element that is more critical to its function than others. The lack of one of these elements in the mother means that a certain organ in the embryo will not develop completely or as it should.

When the baby is born, growth continues, and at this time, inadequate nutrition can further complicate the reflex process discussed here. So can inadequate stimulation. We have all heard the saying, "Before we can learn to walk, we must learn to crawl." If a baby is not allowed to crawl, then his "walking center" in the brain will be held back. If the mother lacks manganese, the "mother love" element, then the child will be hindered in many areas of brain development, learning, and emotional development. A child develops well only in the presence of love. I don't like to say this, but the absence of love is probably as responsible as anything else for laziness, irresponsibility, rebellion, lying, cheating, stealing, and other problems that show lower level functioning of brain faculties in teenagers and adults. It starts in childhood. Love is food for the spirit, mind, and body, and without it, the brain centers and faculties remain incompletely developed and function at lower levels. The child also needs color, music, movement, toys, and attention from the father and mother to develop various faculties and centers normally. These are not "extras," they are basic needs.

In the pediatric ward of one hospital, infants were responding so poorly to treatment that the doctors and nurses had a meeting. They decided to make it a rule that no one could walk through that ward without giving at least one child a hug. As a result, the healing rate in that ward took a dramatic turn for the better. There were fewer deaths, and children were being released at a much faster rate. Love is a brain tonic and a healer.

When I examine the eyes of patients, I sometimes see what are called radii solaris in the iris, spokes that radiate outward from the bowel area of the iris to some part of the body—sometimes the brain. Experience has demonstrated that these spokes reveal the channeling of toxic wastes from the bowel to a particular organ. The toxic material may be carried by the blood, but it is directed to a specific target location just as if it had a map telling it where to go. I believe the map and the reflex that directs the toxins are in the brain.

Hering's law tells us, "All cure comes from the head down, from the inside out, and in reverse order as the symptoms first appeared." Notice, especially, the words "from the head down." Healing is initiated in the brain and mind. It actually begins and proceeds by cleansing of the tissues "from the inside (the bowel) out." When the body and mind are sufficiently strengthened, a healing crisis comes and old toxic deposits and catarrh are thrown off as old symptoms are reexperienced.

It may be that we need to take care of the bowel before we will see any improvement in some of the brain centers and faculties. Nutritional care is not enough when we find a toxic bowel and a toxic bloodstream. We have to take care of these things before good food can bring about rejuvenation and restoration of tissues and functions.

THE POWER OF THE MIND

Doctors know that blood pressure among executives can rise and fall with the stock market. Insomnia is as often the result of a nagging wife or frustrated love, as it is a deficiency of serotonin in the brain. Ulcers, of course, are the reward earned by worriers.

The mind exerts enormous power over the body. Fear can cause the blood to drain from the face, the heart to pound like a drum, the palms of the hands to sweat, the muscles to tremble. Emotional distress can lead to hypertension, allergies, skin eruptions and rashes, peptic ulcers, heart trouble, indigestion, and colitis, not to mention serious mental or nervous breakdowns.

To heal physical problems with origins at the emotional level requires that the emotional problem be released. No doctor can help a patient with arthritis who refuses to give up hate and resentment. No case of ulcers can be permanently healed until the marriage or job problem is taken care of. The asthma and allergies may stay until mother and father give that child the love he or she needs. No one has yet discovered how to heal loneliness and the need for love nutritionally.

Excessive expression of sexuality—the great excitement, passion, stirring of the emotions—can break down the cerebellum. Excessive study and concentration can break down the brain. The executive dilemma, simply put, is that there is a great price to pay, brain-wise, for coping with high responsibilities, stress, important decisions, and critical thinking. Breaking down the cerebellum can produce headaches, loss of ambition, fear of society, and inclination to solitude.

The passive exercises of yoga can do wonders for the nervous system, but we may find out too that we need more rest, more relaxation, more sunshine and fresh air. Skin brushing is good for the nerves. The mountains are good for the nerves, and nature's beauty is a natural nerve tonic.

The sex center of the brain affects other functions as well. I have found that those who have a healthy sex life generally have good circulation, physical vigor, and enthusiasm. These things go together. When the sex center is in balance, all other brain centers tend to be in balance. When it is out of balance, other centers are affected. When we think of the sex center, we have to consider attitudes, beliefs, and the essentials other than sex that make a relationship warm, secure, interesting, and rewarding. Friendship love should precede romantic love in a relationship and should always be there as its foundation. When love is flowing and the sex life is good, the marriage is good, and the appetite and digestion are good. Parsley tea, watermelon seed tea, goat milk, and the iron and sulphur foods are good for balancing and restoring the sex center in the brain.

FEEDING THE MIND AND SPIRIT

The best food for the spirit is truth, and this includes being true to ourselves, our friends, our business associates, and even to our enemies. Do you realize that when we succeed in loving our enemies, they are no longer enemies? My mother used to say, "We need to love others not only for their good but for our own good." This is something to think about.

Truth would not be truth if it only had value in church. Truth must be taken out of the church and put to work at our place of employment, our homes, wherever we go. The higher spiritual ideals in religions feed the spirit and make it strong. I believe it is necessary to nourish the spirit so the spirit can come through the mental and direct us onto the higher paths.

We must realize that we cannot resist and resent and expect to get anywhere in life. Why? Because resistance and resentment—like most negative emotions—cut off the flow of the spirit in our lives. Negative emotions, such as hate, anger, fear, and bitterness are toxic to the spirit and mind. Soul development is blocked or stunted. Brain centers are hindered from opening up. Hate is like a forty-degree-below-zero wind. It freezes virtually everything in its path. Nothing can grow.

Remember, what we put our attention to grows. Do you want to have a strong, capable mind with fully awakened potential? Then you must use the same replacement therapy with the mind that we use with the body. Let the old go; let the new come in. In a healthy mind, as in a healthy body, everything should move and flow, bringing constant renewal. We must do this ourselves and teach it to our patients. Saint Paul said, "Whatever is good . . . whatever is pure . . . think ye on these things." When we put our intention on good, the good grows inside us until it overflows on others. When we put our attention on hate, the same thing happens. I believe we live on what flows out of us. Good is nourishing; love is nourishing; peace and joy are nourishing. Negative thoughts and emotions are toxic to ourselves and to others—much more to ourselves than to others, in fact.

Everything in the mind affects and colors everything else in the mind and body—every cell of the body. What is nourishing to the mind and spirit is nourishing to the body; what is nourishing to the body is nourishing to the mind and spirit. Again, true healing requires that we take the wholistic approach, taking care of body, mind, and spirit. Anything less is not true healing.

REJUVENATING THE MIND—REPLACEMENT THERAPY

Many years ago, Dr. Charlton de Radwan of the University of Vienna gave a series of talks on the use of autosuggestion to renew the mind and its attitudes. His work, of course, is based on the research and discoveries of Emile Coue in France, and I believe much good can be drawn from it.

Suggestion is a powerful tool, and it can be used on oneself or with patients. Dr. de Radwan was once working with a deadly poison in his laboratory, and absentmindedly put a finger in his mouth. Realizing what he had done, he became so sick that an ambulance was called to rush him to the hospital. Within minutes, however, he realized that he had handled the poison only with his other hand—not the one whose finger he had put in his mouth. His symptoms immediately vanished, and he felt fine. The subconscious takes in what we believe, and the body reacts accordingly, which is what makes suggestion so powerful.

We must be very careful in applying suggestion to others. The great danger with suggestion and hypnosis is that if they are used to remove symptoms, or stop a smoking or alcohol habit, other symptoms and problems more severe than the first can come up.

So, we have to be careful. However, we can use this healing tool carefully and productively to bring about certain results safely to patients.

In the case of most disease conditions, we can use suggestion to stimulate positive attitudes, reduce pain, bring about relaxation and better sleep, and reinforce the patient's efforts at carrying out his health regimen conscientiously. When we see that a patient's condition is largely due to psychosomatic or emotional problems, complete regression of all symptoms will come if the patient removes the cause through autosuggestion. I am not saying that suggestion should replace the spiritual things; but we must recognize that the mind and the emotions should be or must be taken care of in some cases before the physical condition will leave. Neurasthenia, compulsion, obsession, fear, anxiety, and perversion are among the conditions that will respond well to suggestion, along with depression, insomnia, spastic colon, colitis, bedwetting, frequent urination, and other mentally-caused problems.

One of the things I have done at the Ranch along this line is to put patients to work in the vegetable garden or at some other form of physical labor, telling them we *earn* good health just as we earn disease. When the mind and body are occupied productively, and the patient believes his health will improve as a result, then it does.

Perhaps the greatest healing comes about when both doctor and patient work as a team, believing in one another and believing in the program designed to take care of whatever condition is involved. You can call it trust, or you can call it faith, but the Bible says, "Faith without works is dead," and I put them to work. The sign in front of the office at my Ranch says, "You're looking for a good doctor—I'm looking for a good patient." Give me a cooperative patient who will listen and follow my instructions faithfully, and you'll find this is the kind of patient who gets well.

Many years ago, I took care of a woman who came to me in a wheelchair. She was almost immobilized with pain, her back curved grotesquely. X-rays showed calcium spurs as big as thumbnails on her spine, and doctors had given up on her. Her attitude was as great a contribution to her healing as the many sodium-rich foods she used. After being completely restored, she said this in front of an audience: "I would have crawled on my hands and knees through Los Angeles to keep my appointments with Dr. Jensen." She believed in me. She believed in what I was doing, and the arthritis and calcium spurs left completely, as verified by new X-rays.

There are times when a sense of financial failure, lack of confidence, loneliness, insecurity, or depression complicates and delays the healing that should be coming in. The following positive affirmations, from Dr. de Radwan, can be given to the patient to bring him out of it. These should be repeated at bedtime, just before going to sleep, with the eyes closed, twenty or thirty times, very quickly.

- *Confidence: Whatever happens, I am calm, capable, and self confident.*
- *Success: Everything I do prospers and brings a wonderful return.*
- *Friendship: I enjoy being with people and helping others.*
- *Happiness: I am content, cheerful, and peaceful, no matter what happens.*
- *Security: I am free, independent, inwardly secure.*

A patient with digestion problems can benefit by saying the following at least five times, one half-hour before meals.

1. *I will digest my food comfortably.*
2. *My digestion is getting stronger.*
3. *My nerves are growing calmer.*
4. *All's well and peaceful in my life.*

Here are some general affirmations that may be repeated twenty or thirty times rapidly before bedtime and upon rising. Select one or more that may be appropriate, and feel free to change the wording so it is more comfortable for you or the patient to speak. Do not allow negative thoughts while speaking these words.

My power within is the fortress of my life. It protects me from all assaults.
I can face reality . . . and I am able to meet any life situation.
I am understanding, cooperative, harmonious.
I am in harmony with myself, with everything around me and nothing brings me out of inner peace.
Everywhere I go I am surrounded by love.

I appreciated Dr. de Radwan's affirmations so much that I created a few of my own:

SERENITY. *My nerves are strong and calm . . . stronger and calmer. I feel in harmony with myself . . . with the universe . . . and with everything around me . . . I am rich with inner powers that give me har-*

mony, security, and serenity . . . Nothing, nobody can bring me out of unity with the Higher Power . . . who protects me from all evils . . . and makes me invincible, invulnerable, unshakable.

NEW VITALITY. *I feel full of health and the joy of living. There is sunshine in my soul today. The clouds have rolled away . . . and I feel confident, reassured, and ever so contented. I feel young, ever so young. Every day in every way I feel younger and younger. I feel like a new and powerful personality, and can overcome everything with the greatest of ease. I feel wonderful . . . simply marvelous.*

The problem with some patients is that they are using some disease condition, organic or psychosomatic, as a "tool" in their relationships. When we believe a lie, we live a lie, and only the truth can bring release from this. For example, a person with inferiority feelings may think he or she is not lovable under normal conditions and is lovable only when sick. To "heal" the inferiority feeling, then, generally releases the dis-ease manifestation. Again, in a bad marriage relationship, either spouse may become ill as a tool to stop the accusations of the other. It is the marriage that needs healing, not the physical condition. Children have been known to manifest allergies, bronchitis, flu symptoms, and many other conditions when they sense they are unloved in the home.

Few doctors manage to avoid the kind of patient, at least now and then, who gives the distinct impression that he or she values a particular disease or condition very highly. It may or may not be possible to help these people, but it is always worth a try. Keep in mind that we can *only* be successful, when dealing with such patients, if they truly believe, consciously and subconsciously, that what we are offering them is better than what they have. This is simply replacement therapy again, plus motivation. For the lonely person or the one with inferiority feelings, genuine friendships can often break them out of it, but they need to first believe they are lovable. Suggestion or affirmation can help with this.

Finally, we may encounter the obstreperous patient whose obsession is to doubt, contradict, or pooh-pooh nearly everything we suggest. It sometimes helps get them going to say, "I'm afraid this program is just a little too tough for you," or "I'm afraid you might even feel great if you did such-and-such." Humor, challenge, and opposition-in-kind can sometimes gain cooperation.

Remember, the mind influences the body, and the problem that originates in the mind can burn out chemical elements just as thoroughly as a problem with a physical basis. Even though the mental problem may be evident to you, nutritional correction is nearly always in order, too.

Here is a short suggestion developed by Dr. de Radwan for presentation before an audience of any size, whose members may have various problems. Before ending your talk or lecture, have a blue light or lights turned on in the room or hall. Tell the audience what you are going to do, and ask them to find a comfortable position and to close their eyes and breathe evenly and deeply. Speak in a soft monotone: *"You are now breathing calmly... deeply... feeling your muscles relax... feel soft heaviness flow through your body. You are now relaxing... relaxing... just as you do before you fall asleep.*

"Remain the way you are, not quite asleep, not quite awake... and imagine that I am speaking directly to your organs... to your liver... to your spleen... to your stomach... to your heart... to your bowel... to your glands... to your brain...

"And, now you feel how the healing forces move freely and automatically through all of you, restoring normal energy and function everywhere, balancing, harmonizing, each with the others, giving and receiving wonderful gifts of healing and well-being, letting the old go, taking on the new...

"And, every day in every way, you are getting better and better..."

After the last word, put on a relaxation record and ask everyone to remain still and relaxed until it is over. When the record has played, turn on a white light or lights.

THOUGHTS ON ANOTHER LEVEL

Just as the biochemical elements are raised vibratorily higher as they evolve up the food chain, so are thoughts and emotions raised vibratorily as they evolve into alignment with eternal truth. Anger has a low vibration that conflicts and creates disharmony in the mind. Anger held in the mind can create mental inflammation. Only eternal truth and higher thoughts should be held in the mind, because they lift the lower vibrations of the body.

If we say, "I am sick," we may be stating a fact, a kind of temporary truth, but it may become a lie by tomorrow or next week. So we say, "I am getting better and better," which remains true even as we get better. Are you staying with me on this? Don't tell others your troubles, unless they are professionals trained to help you, because what we speak affects our minds and bodies vibratorily. When you complain, do you want to establish that dissatisfaction perpetually in your mind? Then why speak of it unless to change it?

Vibrations are the key here. I believe most of us know what lifts us and what tears us down. We know what lifts others and what tears them down. Health comes from the higher vibrations. Wholeness is when the vibrations of all the parts are in harmony and are lifting one another.

It is nowhere more apparent than in studying the brain that health is a way of life; that prayers, thoughts and things so obviously interact at the vibratory level that we must take care of the whole person; and that we must pick the log out of our own eye before we can pick the splinter out of our brother's eye. When we raise our vibrations, we can raise the patient's vibrations—toward wholeness.

CHAPTER 16
Homeopathic Remedies

My introduction to homeopathic work began when I studied with Charles Gesser in Florida many years ago. From him, and later from Drs. Henry Lindlahr and V.G. Rocine, I picked up the knowledge and experience that has helped so much in my own work.

Hering's law of cure, the basis for all my healing work, came from Constantine Hering, a homeopath of the last century. V.G. Rocine, my greatest teacher, was the first to apply homeopathic principles to foods and to the development of the chemical types of man. In my work, I have correlated the chemical basis of foods with iridology and Hering's law to develop an approach to healing through the reversal path and the healing crisis. In other words, my work owes much to homeopathy.

My understanding of vital force and chemical imbalances came out of homeopathy. From my study of homeopathy, I began to realize that whole, pure, and natural foods contain the biochemicals we need, naturally triturated and potentized to meet the needs of the human body perfectly. Many people have been told they need potassium, but they don't realize they can get it from foods that have drawn it out of the earth and transmuted it to a stage fit for human consumption. I believe the homeopath can use foods and get better results than the traditional cell salts offer, because whole, pure, and natural foods not only contain cell salts, but they build new tissue as well. Cell salts can't do that.

WHAT IS HOMEOPATHY?

For those unfamiliar with this healing art, homeopathy had its beginning in the early 1800s, when Samuel Christian Hahnemann, who had studied medicine at Leipzig and Vienna, began searching for a more reliable and effective means of healing than conventional medical practice could offer. His discoveries caught on, and homeopathy spread to all parts of Europe, where it gained acceptance as one of the major healing arts.

Samuel Hahnemann discovered that the same substances that produce a certain set of symptoms in a well person would relieve those same symptoms in a sick person. Quinine, Hahnemann found, would give a well person fever and chills—the same symptoms it so effectively eliminated in malaria victims. He tested many other substances on himself until he had a list of basic remedies. The principle of treatment Hahnemann followed was, *"Similia, similibus curantur,"* which means "Like cures like."

Experimenting with dosage levels, Hahnemann made his most surprising discovery. He found that the more he diluted a remedy, the more powerful and effective it became—just the opposite of what conventional medicine believes. As a result of his early experiments and follow-up studies by successive generations of homeopaths, homeopathic remedies are used in extremely small dosages. Understandably, there are no "undesirable side effects" as we find in so many modern drugs.

The concept behind homeopathy is that everything has an essence or energy pattern permeating and surrounding it. This is natural to the organism, unless disease disrupts it. Hahnemann believed this pattern in people is sustained by the "vital force" that harmonizes mind, soul, and body. The way to cure a person, he believed, was to redirect the vital force to restore the natural pattern in any afflicted organs or tissues. This is what he understood his remedies to be doing. His highly diluted remedies worked because the energy pattern or essence brought into the body interacted with the human energy pattern to restore natural balance.

Remedies are diluted by adding one part of a full-strength cell salt to nine-parts milk sugar or nine parts of an alcohol-distilled water solution. The mixture is "triturated"—combined, shaken, stirred—until the original substance is uniformly distributed through the dilutant. This is the 1X dilution. If made in a one-part-to-ninety-nine-parts ratio, it is known as a 1C dilution. (X is the Roman numeral for ten; C is the Roman numeral for 100.) This process may be repeated to carry the dilution as fine as is desired—30X, 200X or 30C, 200C and so on. It is believed that the effectiveness of highly diluted cell salts is due to their being drawn, through electromagnetic vibrational resonance, directly to the site of inflammation where they are needed.

Remember, these cell salts have all been tested on human subjects to find out what symptoms they bring out in healthy persons. Homeopathy, then, treats symptoms of disease and illness with medicinal substances in highly diluted form that would create these same symptoms in healthy people. And it works. The cell salts find their way to the site of the problem and present the energized or "potentized" chemicals to the tissue in need of them. As the body is strengthened and restored, symptom reversal takes place, and—through a healing crisis—old toxins and catarrh are thrown off. This can happen because deficiencies are being taken care of.

Hering's law of cure says, "All cure starts from the head down, from the inside out and in reverse order as symptoms first appeared." Symptom reversal actually takes place during the healing crisis.

Constantine Hering, the author of this law, studied at the Surgical Academy in Dresden, Germany, and at the University of Leipzig. When he first heard about homeopathy, he was outraged at its unorthodox approach, and decided to expose it as the fraud he believed it must be. However, in researching the subject to discover exactly what sort of fraudulence was involved, he was persuaded instead of its accuracy. He became one of the most well known of the European homeopaths before moving to the United States in 1833.

At the turn of the century, nearly 25 percent of the physicians in the United States were homeopaths. In the past fifty years, however, the influence of homeopathy has dwindled here, and it is not as well received in the United States as it is in Europe, although medical doctors such as Edward Lahn and Henry Lindlahr studied it, took it seriously, and used it along with iridology. Yet, we still find practicing homeopaths here, and most health food stores and some drugstores carry the homeopathic cell salt remedies.

DR. SCHUESSLER'S DISCOVERIES

Every now and then a great pioneer brings something wonderfully new into the healing art. Dr. Wilhelm Henrick Schuessler, a medical doctor and chemist, developed a unique system he called "cellular therapeutics," in which mineral substances called tissue salts or cell salts are used to treat biochemical deficiencies in the body according to homeopathic principles.

Dr. Schuessler did not believe in drugs and suppressants. When treating patients who seemed well fed but were obviously lacking in one or more chemical elements, he came to realize that depleted soils cannot support crops or livestock that will meet our nutritional needs. The missing elements, then, need to be supplied in the diet or disease will intervene. Cellular therapeutics were designed to meet that need.

The human metabolism is constantly in a state of tearing down old cells and building new ones, using nutrients supplied by the blood. If the blood doesn't contain all the right chemicals, we are in trouble. But, even a small amount of any particular element will trigger rebuilding, and bring the body back into harmony.

Health starts at the cell level, as Dr. Schuessler knew. He believed that if we knew which of the basic twelve cell salts were needed, we could take care of the body's basic deficiencies in the chemical elements.

Symptoms whose origins are assumed to be in the cellular metabolism are used to determine which salts are needed. They are: pain, inflammation, constipation, congestion, anemia, catarrh, swelling, bony growths, suppurations, and decay.

The homeopathic remedies, highly diluted (triturated) and potentized (made electrically active by dilution), cannot be compared to the drugs used by Western medicine. Drugs work by interfering with natural physiological processes. Homeopathic remedies work by harmonizing with those processes. Each cell, and each group of similar cells that make up tissue, emit a vibration that attracts certain substances to it and repels others. Disease states change that vibration; chemical deficiencies change it. The homeopathic remedy works because its vibrations are attuned or harmonized very specifically to similar vibrations from metabolically disturbed cell groups, and it circulates through the blood to the precise location where it is needed. When the deficiency is taken care of, the vibration emitted by those cells changes back to normal. Normal cells with adequate supplies of nutrients do not take in the cell salts, and any excess is eliminated from the body.

The highly diluted form of homeopathic cell salts has come under criticism from those who doubt that such a small amount of cell salts can do any good. In health food stores, we find chelated mineral supplements in amounts expressed as milligrams—10, 20, 50, 100 mg, and so on. Why not take these instead? The whole point of the potentized homeopathic remedies lies in the notion that in highly-diluted form, the chemical elements in the remedies are drawn swiftly and specifically to the site of the problem. Once there, the electromagnetic union of the elements with the cells serves a "pump priming" function which stimulates the cells to attract more of the elements they need from the bloodstream. The cells are "potentized" by the arrival of the "potentized" salts. Some homeopaths bring in the idea of essences to explain this rather mysterious effect. However we look at it, the action is basically an energy reaction involving electromagnetic forces and vibrations.

Allergic reactions to homeopathic cell salts are unknown, as are unwanted side effects of any kind. We simply take care of the patient, and the body takes care of its own problems.

How Cell Salts Are Used

I have often said, "Nature cures, but she needs an opportunity." The fundamental principle of health care was summed up very nicely by Dr. William Gull, court physician to Queen Victoria of England, in an address to medical students. "You'll be taught to classify everything, but you'll never be a successful practitioner unless you can cast that tendency behind you. You must never treat a case of pneumonia, but always the person who has it."

Each person is unique. When we use cell salts, we can't simply assign a cell salt to match a specific symptom without considering the individual. The patient's health is made up of many factors.

Inherent weaknesses must be examined. We should listen to the patient's complaint and attempt to trace its source. (Here, iridology is of irreplaceable value.) Besides the twelve basic cell salts developed by Dr. Schuessler, modern research has uncovered many trace elements needed by the body. We must have these, too.

When a cell salt is administered, it may not bring a person to the state of health desired. The elimination of one symptom may disclose another after a week or two. Table 16.1 lists the twelve cell salts, the parts of the body they help, their function, and their deficiency symptoms. Let's take a closer look at the basic cell salts.

Calcium Fluoride (Calc. Fluor.)

Calcium is found mainly in the bones and teeth, but also in the muscles and nerves of the body and in the bloodstream. It is in the walls of blood vessels and in connective tissue. Lack of calcium interferes with proper dentition in infants and has been associated with flabbiness of muscles, a paunchy abdomen, varicose veins, and hemorrhoids. One of calcium's main functions is the preservation of contractile power in elastic tissue. Calcium is necessary whenever there is dilation of the heart and blood vessels; whenever there is prolapsus and displacement of organs; when cracks in the skin, between the fingers and toes, indicate sluggish circulation; when the teeth decay or are found loose in their sockets; and in some cases of obesity. Pain in the tendons or during labor indicates calcium fluoride need. Fluoride is a resistance element, a natural antibiotic; it hardens teeth and bones and stimulates the natural immune system to greater activity. Calcium fluoride is needed when we encounter varicose ulcers, hard chancres, offensively pungent urine, and carbuncles.

Calcium Phosphate (Calc. Phos.)

Without calcium phosphate, there could be no blood coagulation. It has an affinity for albumen; builds up bone tissue; increases gastric juice; and aids in building the dentine of the teeth. It restores tone to weakened organs and tissue. It almost acts as a tonic after debilitating diseases and anemic conditions. This is a very important salt for children, and is used in teething disturbances and delayed dentition. Broken bones do not heal well without this salt. It is one of the best salts for rickets and cases where there may be backwardness and recurring tooth troubles. It is indicated in diphtheria, coldness of the extremities, and albuminuria. It is a great restorative and helps to take care of deep ulcers. It is also helpful in alleviating constant susceptibility to colds, catarrh, phlegm, poor circulation, curvature of the spine, inflammation of the testicles, polyps in the body, sore breasts, and night sweats, and helps to replenish the body's reserves of strength. It works with blood conditions associated with inadequate circulation.

Table 16.1 The Twelve Schuessler Remedies*

Schuessler Cell Salt	Bodily Parts Affected	Function	Deficiency Symptoms
Calc. Fluor. Calcarea Fluorica (Fluoride of Lime)	Bones, elastic tissues, veins, arteries, teeth, joints	Gives tissues the quality of elasticity, preserves contractile power of elastic tissue.	Cracks in the skin, a loss of elasticity, relaxed condition of the veins and arteries, piles, sluggish circulation, loose teeth.
Calc. Phos. Calcarea Phosphoricum (Phosphate of Lime)	Bones, muscles, nerves, brain, connective tissues, teeth	Aids normal growth and development, restores tone and strength, aids digestion, aids bone and teeth formation.	Anemic state of young girls, blood coagulation problems, blood poverty, imperfect circulation, bone weakness, rickets, bronchial asthma.
Calc. Sulph. Calcarea Sulphurica (Sulphate of Lime)	Blood, skin	Blood purifier and healer that removes waste products from the blood. First aid, oxygen carrier, supplementary remedy.	Pimples, sore throat, cold, all conditions arising from impurities in the blood. Congestion, inflammatory pain, high temperature, quickened pulse, lack of red blood corpuscles.
Ferr. Phos. Ferrum Phosphoricum (Phosphate of Iron)	Muscles, nerves, hair, crystalline lens, blood vessels, arteries, red blood cells	First aid, oxygen carrier, supplementary remedy.	Congestion, inflammatory pain, high temperature, rheumatism, quickened pulse, lack of red blood corpuscles, abscesses, bedwetting, fatigue, bronchitis, painful menstruation.
Kali Mur. Kali Muriaticum (Chloride of Potash)	Muscles, blood, saliva	Treats burns, aids digestion, cleanses and purifies the blood.	Sluggish conditions, catarrh, sore throat, torpidity of the liver, white-colored tongue, light-colored stools, coughs, colds, constipation, skin problems.
Kali Phos. Kali Phosphoricum (Phosphate of Potash)	Muscles, nerves, skin	Nerve nutrient, aids breathing, contributes to a contented disposition, sharpens mental faculties.	Nervous headaches, lack of pep, ill humor, skin ailments, nervous asthma, sleeplessness, depression, timidity, tantrums, poor concentration.

*Reprinted with the permission of NuAge Laboratories Ltd., St. Louis, Missouri.

Schuessler Cell Salt	Bodily Parts Affected	Function	Deficiency Symptoms
Kali Sulph. Kali Sulphuricum (Sulphate of Potash)	Skin, intestine, hair, stomach, tissue cells	Oxygen-carrier, anti-friction, maintains hair, benefits perspiration and respiration.	Boxed-in feeling, intestinal disorders, stomach catarrh, inflammatory conditions, eruptions on the skin and scalp with scaling, shifting pains.
Mag. Phos. Magnesia Phosphoricum (Phosphate of Magnesia)	Muscles, nerves, bones	Antispasmodic, benefits the nervous system, helps ensure rhythmic movement of muscular tissue.	Menstrual pains, stomach cramps, flatulence, neuralgia, neuritis, sciatica, headaches with darting stabs of pain, cramps, muscular twitching.
Nat. Mur. Natrum Muriaticum (Chloride of Soda)	Cartilage, mucous cells, glands	Water distributor, aids nutrition and glandular activity, aids cell division and normal growth, aids digestion.	Low spirits, headaches with constipation, thin/watery blood, heartburn, toothache, hay fever, craving for salt and salty foods, weak eyes.
Nat. Phos. Natrum Phosphoricum (Phosphate of Soda)	Nerves, muscles, joints, digestive organs	Acid neutralizer, aids in the assimilation of fats and other nutrients.	Stiffness and swelling of the joints, acidic blood condition, rheumatism, lumbago, worms, golden-yellow coating at the root of the tongue.
Nat. Sulph. Natrum Sulphuricum (Sulphate of Soda)	Liver	Eliminates excess water, ensures adequate bile, removes poison-charged fluids, treats rheumatic ailments.	Influenza, humid asthma, malaria, liver ailments, brownish-green coating of the tongue, bitter taste in the mouth.
Silica Silicic Oxide (Pure Silica)	Connective tissues, skin, nerves	Cleanser and eliminator, initiates the healing process, insulator of the nerves, restores the activity of the skin.	Smelly feet and armpits, pus formation, abscesses, boils, styes, tonsillitis, brittle nails, stomach pains, diseases affecting bone surfaces, skin ailments.

Calcium Sulphate (Calc. Sulph.)

This is considered the salt of blood purification and is a healer. It is especially indicated in liver troubles, which so many people have when they are sick or have used alcohol to excess. It is part of the liver cells. Because the liver takes care of worn-out cells, we need calcium sulphate—otherwise, the destruction and disposal of these worn-out cells is delayed. It is particularly indicated where we have old fistula abscesses in the body, and it is great for preventing suppuration indicated in dysenteries that have become chronic. It helps to cause tissues to discharge their contents readily, throwing off decaying organic matter. It helps remove dormant, decaying material that can destroy or injure surrounding tissue. It is indicated in conditions arising from impurities in the bloodstream. It is specific in aborting gum boils. This salt is beneficial for elderly people suffering from neuralgia and headaches with nausea; for catarrh, acne, and pimples that occur in adolescence; and for abscesses and wounds that will not heal readily and tend to become septic. It is helpful when a person gets sensitive and touchy; when a sore throat is developing; or when a cold is coming on.

Iron Phosphate (Ferr. Phos.)

This is one of the great cell salts. It is the oxygen carrier in the body. It is found in the makeup of hemoglobin. Iron helps take up the oxygen from the air as we inhale it into the lung structure. It helps improve the vital force that sustains life within us. Many times this ferric phosphate, working in hand with potassium sulphate, helps carry oxygen in greater abundance to the cell structures within the blood vessels. This is a great supplementary remedy for inflammatory pains, high temperatures, quickened pulse, and congestion. Whatever the problem, it always calls for more oxygen. This particular salt should be used in the first stages of any disease until the inflammatory symptoms subside. It is a first aid remedy in hemorrhages. There is hardly any illness where ferric phosphate could not be used to advantage. It is a wonderful remedy, especially with children, for prevention of constipation and diarrhea. It takes care of debility and listlessness, bleeding wounds, cuts, and abrasions. In advancing years, it is most frequently needed. Ferric phosphate can be used in mechanical injuries and the first stages of any disease or inflammation such as peritonitis, meningitis, bronchitis, and the first stages of fevers and congestions. It is indicated in teething, fever, hemorrhoids, inflamed rectal conditions, nose bleeds, children who retain urine, uterine hemorrhages, and bleeding from any part of the body, including excessive menses. This is in no sense an iron tonic. Its actions are entirely nutritional without any side effects.

Potassium Chloride (Kali Mur.)

This cell salt is the remedy for sluggish conditions in the body. It combines with organic substances and fibrin. Whenever there is catarrh and other symptoms affecting the skin and mucous membranes, the patient should be using Kali Muriaticum (potassium chloride). Whenever there is any irritation under the skin, and there is a raising of small blisters or papules, this salt is indicated. This, of course, occurs in smallpox. Potassium chloride unites with hydrogen to form the hydrochloric acid for digestion. Kali Mur. should be used in all cases of inflammatory or catarrhal conditions, and where white-coated tongue and a light-colored stool show a lack of bile and torpidity of the liver. It is also recommended for coughs, colds, tonsillitis, bronchitis, sore throats; and children's ailments such as measles, chickenpox, rheumatic fever, shingles, asthma, gastric derangements, scurvy, acne, and where there are soft swellings, as in mumps. It is needed in the production of saliva and in the early stages of digestion, when symptoms develop from eating fatty or rich foods and when there is a lack of appetite. This tissue salt is useful as a first aid for the treatment of burns.

Potassium Phosphate (Kali Phos.)

This is a nerve nutrient. It is effective in treating neurotic disorders, neurasthenias, and most paralytic conditions. It helps maintain a happy, contented disposition and sharpens the mental faculties. Kali Phos. is a constituent of all the fluids and tissues of the body, especially the gray matter of the brain and nerves. It is in muscles, blood cells, and plasma. People can develop anxiety, ill humor, bashfulness, and timidity, and even laziness and tantrums may be regarded as Kali Phos. symptoms. The saponification of fat is aided by the presence of Kali Phos., and it is a pick-me-up for the nervous system. It is also good for people who complain about nerves and irritating skin ailments such as shingles, offensive secretions and excretion, uterine hemorrhages, nerve depression, melancholia, mania, hysteria, suicidal thoughts, despair, sexual impotence, a lack of nerve and mental powers, a muscular wasting, delirium, nervous asthma, squinting, giddiness, twitching, some nightmares, some phobias, fear of light, and fear of open spaces.

Potassium Sulphate (Kali Sulph.)

Internal breathing of the tissues depends upon Kali Sulph. It works especially well with the mucous membranes that line the internal organs. When in combination with Kali Sulph. and Ferric Phos., it is the great carrier of oxygen to the cells and tissues. It is indicated where there is a yellowish discharge from the skin and mucous membranes. A deficiency causes chilliness, flashes of heat, weariness, heaviness, anxieties, fear, sadness, giddiness, and palpitation. It helps to maintain the hair in a healthy state, and rids scaling on the scalp and skin. It helps alleviate pains in the limbs, especially indicated in the chronic stage of inflammation. It is effective with intestinal catarrh, albuminuria, and jaundice; it may relieve fullness in the pit of the stomach, peeling of the lips, chilliness, fleeting pains in the joints, stomach catarrh, and it promotes perspiration during inflammatory conditions. It is appropriate when we have symptoms that are worse in the evening.

Magnesium Phosphate (Mag. Phos.)

This is known as the antispasmodic tissue salt. It is necessary to ensure rhythmic and coherent movement throughout the body. When the white nerve fibers contract causing spasms and cramps, Mag. Phos. is necessary and is quick to relieve pain, especially cramping, shooting, darting, or spasmodic pains. The function of the white matter in the brain and nerves is dependent chiefly upon Mag. Phos. It helps those who have a highly nervous temperament, are generally exhausted, or are too tired to stand up or to sit down. Magnesium phosphate is necessary to allay sciatica, neuritis, headaches, neuralgia, nerve pains; and relieves muscular twitching, hiccoughs, cramps, ovarian neuralgia, constipation in infants, colicky pain, spasms of the bladder, convulsive fits of coughing, dysmenorrhea, nervous asthma, epilepsy, menstrual pains, stomach cramps, and flatulence. Spasmodic shivering, fits, profuse perspiration, stammering, barber's itch, and dyspepsia have been helped by magnesium phosphate.

Sodium Chloride (Nat. Mur.)

Nat. Mur. is a water-distributing tissue salt. It is the watery solution from Nat. Mur. that gives us the power of dissolving biochemical salts in the fluids of the body. It helps break up the insoluble phosphates of lime. Its prime function is to maintain a proper degree of moisture throughout the body. Division in normal growth could not proceed without this tissue salt. It is closely associated with glandular activity and the internal secretions that play such an important part in the physiological process. When we have excessive moisture or excessive dryness in any part of the body, Nat. Mur. shows up as a deficiency. It is a constituent of every liquid and solid in the body, and carries water to the tissue cells. Waterlogging can result if we do not have sufficient Nat. Mur. The patient then feels bloated, heavy, chilly, drowsy, and has watery eyes. He feels languid, salivation appears, and he experiences low spirits. The blood thins and becomes watery, and the skin becomes pale. There may be difficult stools, with rawness and soreness of the anus, headaches with constipation, feeling of hopelessness, heavy, watery mucus and discharges, sneezing, dry, painful nose and throat symptoms, fermentation with slow digestion, craving for salt, toothache, facial neuralgia, the flow of tears, hay fever, drowsiness with muscular weakness, chafing of the skin, unrefreshing sleep, tiredness in the morning, aftereffects of alcohol stimulants, loss of taste and smell, craving of salt and salty foods. An important function of Nat. Mur. is the production of hydrochloric acid. Too little acid means slow digestion, especially of calcium-rich food. It is needed in vomiting of watery mucus; mumps with salivation; chronic constipation due to dryness; watery blisters anywhere, such as in Herpes Zoster, especially on face and lips; winter cough; fluttering; periodic attacks of gout—sciatica, and numbness of the hands and feet. Remember, approximately two-thirds of your body is composed of water. Hence, a vital role is played by Nat. Mur., the water distributor, in all the life processes.

Sodium Phosphate (Nat. Phos.)

Nat. Phos. is an acid neutralizer that helps tremendously in all ailments arising from an acid condition of the blood. It is a great remedy for the so-called acid-diathesis. It is also important for the proper functioning of the digestive organs; the assimilation of fats and other nutrients is dependent upon the action of this remedy. A deficiency of Nat. Phos. allows uric acid to form salts that finally develop into joint stiffness, swelling, and other rheumatic symptoms. Nat. Phos. is indicated for a golden yellow or creamy coating at the root of the tongue, dyspepsia caused by fatty foods, or sleeplessness caused by indigestion. This salt has power to take up peptones and emulsify fats, and aids acute articular rheumatism, and gout. Used for sour breath and conjunctivitis, it is also recommended for rheumatism; fibrocysts; lumbago, and associated ailments such as leukorrhea, soreness of intercostal muscles; pains in knees, ankles, and balls of the feet; and when legs give way from weakness.

Sodium Sulphate (Nat. Sulph.)

Nat. Sulph. regulates the density of the intercellular fluids. It functions to cleanse the tissue cells by eliminating excess water.

Nat. Sulph is a great remedy for constipation and biliousness. It is indicated in the treatments affecting the liver and sandy deposits in the urine, as well as watery infiltrations in a brownish-green coating of the tongue and a bitter taste in the mouth. It ensures an adequate supply of free-flowing healthy bile so necessary for the later stages of digestion. It relieves bilious vomiting and diarrhea, influenza, edema, vomiting and diarrhea, bilious irritability. Nat. Sulph. is effective for mental troubles caused by injury to the head, diabetes, painter's colic, appendicitis, liver and kidney disorders, and gallbladder problems. In conditions arising that allow waste fluids to accumulate in the blood and tissues in autointoxication, Nat. Sulph. ensures the disposal of these poisonous fluids. It is important in the treatment of rheumatic ailments, as well as ringing of the ears. It is indicated for the following: large prostate gravel; morning sickness in pregnancy; bronchial catarrh; edema of feet and ankles; awakening at night with an attack of asthma; warts around the eyes, scalp, face, chest, neck, anus, and so forth; and humid asthma. Malaria and other conditions associated with humidity need this remedy. A few doses of Nat. Sulph. will help to dispel that languid feeling so often experienced during a spell of humid, oppressive weather.

Silicon Oxide (Silica)

This salt is a cleanser and an eliminator, and is found in nature as quartz and flint from which glass is made, and in the hardness in straw, bamboo, and certain grasses. It is also responsible for the stiffness found in the covering of brans and cereal grains. All whole grains are high in silica. It initiates healing by promoting suppuration and breaking up pathological accumulations such as abscesses. Silica is found in the hair, nails, epidermis, and the surfaces of the bones and connective tissues. It is therefore one of the great elements needed for the action of the brain, spinal cord, and nerves; it helps form the myelin sheath which insulates nerves. It restores the activity of the skin by aiding in cleansing. When the feet do not perspire properly, silica can help. Whenever we have suppression of any kind in the body, silica seems to open it up and start the elimination process. It is indicated for offensive perspiration of the feet and underarms and when the system is irritable, weak, and the nerve supply is lowered. When we have exaggerated reflexes, we should think of silica. When a person is cranky, oversensitive to noise, and absent-minded, silica is indicated. It is effective for curing sweating at night, especially of head and neck. It can be used for cerebral apoplexy, headaches from hunger, styes, eye discharges, or when the corners of the mouth ulcerate. Silica is recommended for chronic neuritis, itching of the rectum, thickening of nasal mucous membranes, boils and carbuncles, encysted tumors, large, bloated abdomen in children, cracked nipples, ulcerated chronic bronchitis, hip joint disease, ingrown toenails, and weak ankles. It is especially good in tonsillitis when pus begins to form.

Chemical Balances

Some chemists claim that sodium balances calcium. Magnesium also balances calcium. Fluorine balances calcium. Iodine balances calcium. Calcium balances nitrogen. Sodium balances potassium. Iodine balances carbon. Magnesium balances phosphorus. Sulphur balances phosphorus. Manganese balances fluorine. Nitrogen balances oxygen. Chlorine balances hydrogen.

A lack of cell salts in body chemistry creates an imbalance in the body, as we have stated. Cell salts, as Dr. Schuessler developed them, enter the blood in the form of electrically-charged ions. They are able to go through the cell membranes by osmosis. It is not necessary for them to go through the digestive process. They are prepared in minute dosages; the more they are diluted, the more powerful the effect upon the body. In acute cases, the cell salts are best dissolved in water, about nine tablets in a tumbler three-fourths full of water. Take just a sip or a mouthful every quarter to half hour. In subacute cases, the less urgent cases, take three tablets every two or three hours, slowly dissolved on the tongue.

In chronic or old-standing cases: Take three tablets daily. Acute symptoms and subacute symptoms: Use thirty to two hundred potency in frequent repetition, like every twelve or twenty-four hours. In less chronic symptoms, every four to six hours, or every twelve hours.

CHEMICAL VERSUS BIOCHEMICAL

Whenever we go to the health food store, we find organic fruits and vegetables in the bins. Organic, in this case, means grown naturally, without chemical fertilizers, sprays, artificial coloring, waxing, and so forth. Most people understand this. But, technically, the term organic refers to a carbon-based compound found in living matter, and the drug companies know how to manufacture many such compounds directly from inorganic chemicals. Inorganic chemicals are those found in the earth, or those which can be extracted and refined from the earth. They are not "live" in any sense of the word.

All things—biochemical, organic, and inorganic—are made of chemical elements. There isn't anything on the physical plane that isn't chemical. Air is a mixture of chemical gases. Water is hydrogen, oxygen, and whatever other chemicals happen to be dissolved in it. The earth and everything on it is made of chemicals.

A biochemical is an element or compound in or taken from a living thing—plant, animal, or whatever. Plants take the chemical elements from the soil and turn them into biochemicals by the power of sunlight and photosynthesis. We can take a plant like wheat, mill it, grind it to a fine flour, and bleach it, and the process renders it from a "live" biochemical food to a "dead" organic food. It is still organic—not inorganic—but it is lifeless, dead, and unfit for human consumption.

The difference between chemicals and biochemicals is that biochemicals have life energy that we can use. We are vibratory beings, and we cannot exist without the vibration of live biochemicals that come to us through plant and animal life. We cannot live on inorganic chemicals—they must be biochemical. Biochemical means life-giving. It has the life force in a vibratory state that is different from the material state of the atoms and molecules, different even from the electrical state of the inorganic chemicals. It harmonizes and comes up to the vibratory force that the human being needs. We do not have the capability to transmute the "raw" chemical elements into living biochemicals that are suitable for use by the human body, which is why man looks to the pure, whole, and natural foods of the plant kingdom and some foods from the animal kingdom.

We need biochemical foods. We can do without the rest. Understanding these distinctions is important. A food or supplement can be organic and still be worthless—but if it is *biochemical* it is probably all right. One further thing: A fruit or vegetable may be fresh, biochemical, and "organic," but it may also have been grown on depleted soil, and thus be deficient in essential biochemical nutrients (such as calcium) that we need for good health. We need to shop wisely. Ask questions about the food you buy. Find out where it was grown and by whom. Let the produce buyers in the stores know that you are interested more in quality than in appearance.

The difference between biochemical and inorganic is dramatically illustrated in the example of one of my patients who came to the Ranch with a severe calcium deficiency and several leg ulcers oozing pus. She had been to several of the top medical clinics in the United States, where doctors diagnosed her as calcium deficient and prescribed an inorganic calcium supplement. It didn't work. Her body could not absorb the inorganic calcium, which was not much different from chalk. I knew the sun controlled calcium, so I instructed her in how to prepare a juice from finely chopped green vegetable tops. (This was before the days of juicers.) She would soak the chopped greens in water, then strain the liquid through cheesecloth and drink it. The ulcers were healed within a few weeks. Inorganic chemicals are potentized, altered in their vibratory rate as they are assimilated into the living protoplasm of plants. They are much more compatible with the needs of the human body.

NATURE AND HOMEOPATHY

V.G. Rocine was a Norwegian homeopath. He knew about cell salts, trituration, potentization, and proper dosages, but he pioneered a new way.

Rocine brought out the fact that in natural foods and herbs, the biochemical salts are there, naturally triturated and potentized by Nature, by sunshine and photosynthesis, by the slow movement of water and soil minerals into the root system, and by the natural processes of enzymatic action and chelation in the leaves and roots of each plant. As God made these plants for man, He designed the fruits, vegetables, and herbs to have the proper trituration.

Carrots have sodium and potassium, but in what proportion? As we use the natural foods in variety, we find the proper proportion is there. We find from experience that a balance is taking place in the body, so we know the proportions are right.

I have followed V.G. Rocine's methods of using natural, pure, and whole foods in place of homeopathic cell salts for many decades in my sanitarium work. I have watched symptoms disappear. I have seen Hering's law of cure at work. Healing crises came, bringing out the chronic lesions, suppurations, boils, suppressed conditions of childhood. I knew I was reversing the problems as they had come to the body, and it was evident that the cell salt activity was taking place in the body.

Using iridology, I found healing lines, fine white trabeculae, coming into the dark lesions of the iris as the tissues of the body were cleansed and renewed. When these lines became acute and white, raised up in the iris stroma, I knew that a healing crisis was approaching, and it always came. I could see in the iris the progress from degenerative to chronic, chronic to subacute, subacute to acute. Patients confirmed these findings by noticing that their symptoms were leaving.

The foods we used were compatible with all of the natural, drugless methods—the water treatments, exercise, color, fresh air, and sunshine. By taking care of the inside of the body, we could see signs of healing coming on the outside of the body, just as we had predicted and expected. Of course, it took a great deal of experience and a considerable number of years for me to learn these things. To learn to translate from symptoms to the causes of those symptoms is an art that comes only with time, discipline, training, and experience.

I look at the human body as we might look at parsley growing in the soil. Give it the right nutrients, the right biochemicals, the right amount of sunshine and water, and it will grow to be healthy and disease-free. But, it must be done Nature's way. I am convinced there is a "parsley principle" within us, a godly principle by which all the cells of the body will select exactly the nutrients they need from the bloodstream, provided that we eat the right foods. It is in this way that natural health and harmony are developed.

It never occurred to me to learn the medical terminology for the diseases, conditions, and various physiological processes underlying them, except as they came to me in what I read or encountered in sanitarium work. I don't need to know the name of a disease if I can discover what has caused it and can help the patient eliminate that cause. Classification and technical terminology cannot heal or aid in healing. Iridology reveals tissue inflammation levels, not symptoms or diseases. No doubt, there is some correlation between the system of classification of Western medicine and the findings of iridology. The future will tell.

Meanwhile, it is obvious that both Western medicine and iridology have much more to learn. Both are incomplete, unfinished. I don't think, however, that any healing art or science is complete in itself. Each needs the others.

To me, homeopathy is at its best when applied through nutrition and guided by iridology. The combination of inorganic chemicals in plants by Nature to form the higher evolved vibratory forms of cell salts is the best way to go. Man can give Nature a hand, but he cannot outdo her. Nature knows best.

CHAPTER 17

Helping a Patient
Reach His Potential

Toxic accumulations in the body affect all organs, and chemical deficiencies break down inherently weak organs. No one has a body that is working at 100 percent of its potential. Those who suffer from chronic disease are only working at about 40 percent of their potential. In the subacute stage, the efficiency and motivation of every organ of the body are impaired. The health potential is usually down around 20 percent in the subacute stage. Eighty percent of all patients who are being treated by doctors are in the chronic stage, so these patients are 40 percent potential-poor. We must learn to raise this potential.

THREE STEPS TOWARD RAISING POTENTIAL

The first step toward reaching 100 percent potential is cleaning out catarrh, toxic settlements, and residues of drugs in the tissues. These accumulations are triggering many symptoms, weakening the tissues and encouraging the development of chronic disease. The patient's potential level of health is lowered, so we must cleanse him of these toxic accumulations.

The sources of these unwanted substances in the body are food, water, air, cosmetics, and drugs. Chemical taints are also inherited from parents and grandparents. The person affected by these inherited taints is called the *medeic* person. The medeic person is one who has gone from one doctor to another, one cure to another, tried different diets and drugs, and is developing a list of symptoms that don't respond to treatment. The immunity of this kind of person is broken down, and he has difficulty overcoming sickness.

The second thing the iridologist must do is to determine the nutritive requirements, functional ability, and chemical deficiency of every organ. He should explore the inherent background of the patient. These factors determine how well the immune system will function in preventing disease.

Once the nutritive requirements and chemical deficiencies of the patient are determined, the iridologist should design a diet for the patient. This diet should include all of the nutrients that are deficient in the patient's organs. Of course, the patient must cooperate fully with the iridologist by following the diet closely.

The third thing the iridologist must do is revive the nervous system. A healthy nervous system is so important. This system carries impulses to and from the brain. Stress, fear, and excessive emotion can damage the nervous system and prevent the body from working up to its potential. When the nerves are overstressed, mineralization breaks down and produces deficiencies in our inherently weak organs.

To repair any part of the brain and nervous system, we should rest for a while. Recreation, relaxation, and humor will help repair the brain. The brain and nervous system take four times longer to repair and rebuild than any other tissue in the body. They must be fed properly. If they are not, the brain and nerve paths will not function correctly. When this happens, the brain is unable to supervise bodily functions as it should, and we become vulnerable to mental and physical disease and abnormalities. It is extremely important, because of this, to take proper care of the brain and nerves at all times.

As we put these factors together, they begin to shed light on the processes that lead to a disease and offer a profile of the health level. A disease is a condition involving various organs and the systems connected with those organs. The iridologist does not treat a disease, but he does treat the person who has the symptoms. Determining what stage the patient may be in will tell the iridologist what healing steps are necessary.

THE WHOLISTIC APPROACH

Once the level of health has been reached through the use of whole, pure, natural foods, it can be maintained through the wholistic approach. The wholistic approach states that every part of the body must work together harmoniously. What affects one organ affects every organ.

Those who practice iridology believe in preventive medicine. This is also in line with all health practitioners who follow the wholistic approach.

Those who follow the wholistic approach to healing believe that health should be maintained on a daily basis. The nerve force and metabolic energies of the body should be released, and the elimination channels should be kept open. The body should be receiving the nutrients from a healthy diet of whole foods, so that every organ will be operating at 100 percent of its potential. This is how the body should be cared for—it should be treated properly *before* any symptoms of disease arise. Each organ contributes to the well-being of every other organ, and each organ should be taken care of.

The person who eats whole, pure, natural foods will maintain his level of health. A positive philosophy of life will help maintain this optimum level. Avoidance of harmful chemicals, food additives, pollution, and drugs is also important. Fresh air and exercise should be a part of the life of anyone who wishes to maintain high health potential.

COMMON CONDITIONS IN PATIENTS

Below is list of conditions that I believe nearly everyone has. I have developed these statistics after examining thousands of patients. Many of these symptoms can be hidden or preclinical, but they are evident to the iridologist. These statistics are evidence that very few people have any organ that is working at 100 percent of its potential.

- Nearly everyone who comes into my office as a patient has a 20 percent underactivity in the metabolic processes of the body.
- Most of my patients have a 50 percent underactivity caused by toxic settlements acting as an infection in the elimination channels, especially the bowels.
- There is a 20 percent mineral deficiency in every person who comes into the office.
- There is a 20 percent ignorance about the laws of food that we must follow in order to balance our diet.
- In 40 percent of the patients, there is an imbalance in the endocrine system and sexual system.
- There is a 25 percent brain anemia in almost everyone who comes into the office. This is very important to see, because the brain is the source of motivation and activity for the rest of the organs.
- With the extreme amount of acidity and catarrh that follows every disease in the body, we find a 25 percent loss of function in the lymph glands and lymph organs such as the spleen. This means the electrolytes must be restored, and the lymphatic system must be built up.
- One hundred percent of these patients have bowel trouble.
- One hundred percent have poor skin elimination.
- Ninety percent have kidney underactivity or a deterioration beginning to settle in that particular organ.
- One hundred percent of the people who come in have an underactive digestive system.
- One hundred percent have a mineral deficiency in the stomach wall—a lack of hydrochloric acid or an overactive secretion of hydrochloric acid. The average stomach balance runs to an 80 percent lack of hydrochloric acid, and probably only 15 percent have an excess of hydrochloric acid.

- One hundred percent of the Animation and Life Center of the brain is affected, which brings on fatigue. This center is where will and the fire of life originate.
- One hundred percent have at least six to eight inherent weaknesses. Many have as many as twenty-five, and sometimes more.

IRIDOLOGY EVALUATES THE EFFECTIVENESS OF EACH HEALING ART

The advanced iridologist is most effective in ensuring that good health comes to the patient. He has the opportunity of observing the eyes and making constant improvements in his patient's body activities. The iridologist does his patient a favor by giving him a new outlook, and by giving the body new tissue to work with. As one system improves, all other systems will benefit.

There will be times when the patient will be treated by other practitioners of the healing arts while he is seeing the iridologist. The iridologist can work with these practitioners to help his patient reach his potential. By examining the iris he can see the extent of healing that is going on in the patient's body.

The chiropractor or acupuncturist can see that their patients have energy flowing through every meridian, every organ in the body. This energy is similar to the quickening effect that comes when toxic materials are cleansed from the body. This may also be accomplished when massage, exercise, and manipulation break up tension and fixation, energy blocks that are having a deteriorating effect on the body and health. Other methods that can help are water treatments, air therapy, and psychological therapy. Each organ, gland, bone, nerve, and brain center is helped by each of these therapies, because the body is a community of interrelated structures. There are quickening methods, elimination methods, and new tissue replacement methods that can repair damaged tissue. Then, old, damaged tissue can be replaced by new.

Occasionally, doctors encounter extremes, such as a man interviewed on television who weighed over 1,000 pounds. He couldn't even get out of his house! He had only one bowel movement every sixty days. Think of going without a bowel movement for two months! He has now been put on a high-fiber reducing diet, but it is hard to believe he is still alive. This man is under the care of doctors now, and this is just the kind of situation where iridology could be such a help. Using iridology, the most underactive, toxic, and chemically deficient organs could be seen. The iridologist could work with other health practitioners, and they could all work together to help the patient reach his health potential.

Those who follow the drugless health arts do not work for a disease cure. Instead, we work for an energy buildup of all organs in the body, so those affected by the disease will cast off septic encumbrances, aided by the supportive strength of all other organs in the body. This process will build up weak organs and enable them to reach the highest level of function possible.

In advanced iridology, there is the opportunity to help all the different healing professions by showing where the problems are in the body. Then, the iridologist can determine what kind of nutritional support will give the best assistance to the therapy being used.

The main advantage of advanced iridology is that it can help build a health level that is the highest possible. Health seems almost impossible to achieve in this day of disease and environmental degeneration. However, it is to our great advantage to have as much health as possible and as little disease as possible. This is the great potential of iridology in its advanced application.

Afterword

There is more research needed in iridology. When we do not have a complete art or science to work with, we should, at least, be prepared to be open-minded about future developments.

The average iridologist is a person of compassion who wants his patients to have a better life. There are really no "bad" people working in iridology. Most of the people who work in iridology are idealists who have a calling to do the better things in life. With that calling and with the help that nature can give those who follow its laws, iridologists should be able to accomplish a good deal in the healing arts.

We can shorten the time it takes to get rid of some of the health problems that we are working with today by using iridology and nutrition. They form a natural "team" which helps prevent disease, build health, and give you a longer life, a life that has energy, hope, and power. Iridology and nutrition can help the elderly live a good life. The elderly shouldn't have to be on drugs or have organ transplants or live in convalescent homes.

We in iridology owe humanity a humane, compassionate program of health care. The greatest morality will come from following nature as much as we possibly can. Nature is the healer.

Today there is a tremendous increase in disease, but there are few answers for many problems. I don't say iridology, if used more widely, would solve everything, but it would certainly bring a giant step forward for mankind in the health arts.

A Creed for Iridology

We believe in iridology as the "eye" of the natural healing arts, the window through which the wholistic perspective on health becomes understandable.

We believe in iridology as a reliable means of assessing what is happening in the body. When we know what is happening in the body, we can choose the appropriate therapy leading to high-level wellness.

We believe in iridology as the analysis of choice to use in any of the healing arts to monitor and evaluate how well a therapy is working.

We believe in iridology as the only analysis which reveals abnormal tissue conditions before symptoms appear and shows abnormal conditions for which no symptoms will ever appear.

We believe in iridology as a wonderful means of demonstrating the rewards of choosing a healthy way of life, the ideal of preventive medicine.

We believe in iridology and nutrition as the twin guiding stars that will usher in a new profession that is equally uplifting for both doctor and patient.

_____

Signature

Index

About the Author

Bernard Jensen was born March 25, 1908, in Stockton, California. Following in his father's footsteps, he entered the West Coast Chiropractic College in Oakland, California at the age of 18. Shortly after his graduation, his health failed. Doctors diagnosed the problem as bronchiectasis, a severe and often fatal lung condition for which there was no known cure. He was told that medical science could offer him no hope.

Unwilling to give up, young Dr. Jensen sought the help of a Seventh-Day Adventist physician who taught him the basics of proper nutrition, pulled him off all "junk" foods, and placed him on a natural food diet. Improvement was slow, but steady. As a result of a breathing exercise program developed by Thomas Gaines, he added four inches to his chest in a year's time. Because nature offered him a cure when medical science could do nothing, Dr. Jensen determined to learn all he could about natural healing.

His training included postgraduate courses at the National Chiropractic College in Chicago, Illinois. Later, Dr. Jensen returned to California to study iridology, the science of interpreting tissue conditions from the iris, with Dr. R.M. McLain at the International School of Arts and Sciences in San Francisco, California.

To expand his knowledge of health work, Dr. Jensen studied bowel care with Dr. John Harvey Kellogg of Battle Creek, Michigan, and Dr. Max Gerson of New York, the latter known for his use of nutrition, diets, supplements, and enemas in the treatment of degenerative disease. Among others, Dr. Jensen also studied with Dr. O.B. Shellberg of New York, a colonics specialist; Dr. Ralph Benner, of the Bircher-Benner Clinic in Switzerland; Dr. John Tilden of Denver, Colorado; and Dr. George Weger of Redlands, California.

Dr. Jensen operated several health sanitariums in California, the first in Ben Lomond, the second at Alta Dena, and the last at Escondido. It is this last sanitarium that he refers to as "the Ranch." At the sanitariums, he lived with his patients day in and day out. "The sanitarium was my university," Dr. Jensen says, "and patients were in my books." The sanitariums were living laboratories where he was able to observe firsthand what best brought patients back to health.

Over the years, Dr. Jensen has received many honors and awards, including Knighthood in the Order of St. John of Malta; the Dag Hammarskjold Peace Award of the Pax Mundi Academy in Brussels, Belgium; and an award from Queen Juliana of the Netherlands for his nutritional work. In 1982, he also received the National Health Federation's Pioneer Doctor of the Year award.

At the age of 76, Dr. Jensen earned his Ph.D. from the University of Humanistic Studies in San Diego, California, climaxing a lifetime of study, work, and teaching in the healing arts. He has lectured in 55 countries around the world and has authored over 40 books on the subjects of natural health care and iridology.

Now in his eighties, Dr. Jensen continues to write, lecture, travel, and learn.

If You've Enjoyed Reading This Book . . .

. . . why not tell a friend about it? If you're interested in learning more about Dr. Bernard Jensen's approach to health, here are some other titles you may find to be informative, engaging, and fun.

Vibrant Health From Your Kitchen

A warm and wonderful tour through Dr. Jensen's latest discoveries about food, nutrition, and health, this book provides the guidance needed to keep your family disease-free, healthy, and happy.

Tissue Cleansing Through Bowel Management

Toxin-laden tissue can become a breeding ground for disease. This remarkable book instructs you in the removal of toxins and the restoration of health and youthfulness through the cleansing and care of the organs of elimination.

Food Healing for Man

We now know that foods can repair the tissue damage that accompanies most illness and disease. Look over the shoulders of the great pioneer nutritionists as they investigate the links between nutrition and disease.

Chlorella: Gem of the Orient

Why does Dr. Jensen consider chlorella—a green alga—the most valuable broad-spectrum food supplement discovery of the twentieth century? You'll find out in this unusually beautiful, fully illustrated, hard cover book.

Creating a Magic Kitchen

This is Dr. Jensen's introductory primer on the art of selecting and preparing foods for the best of health. Short, easy to understand, and handy to use, this is the perfect book for anyone who wants a more healthful and enjoyable lifestyle.

Nature Has a Remedy

This popular classic provides a delightful description of the many paths to natural healing—foods, herbs, exercise, climate selection, personology, and hundreds of effective remedies.

World Keys to Health and Long Life

Based on Dr. Jensen's travels to over fifty-five countries, this fascinating book describes the health and longevity secrets of centenarians interviewed in the Hunza Valley of India; Vilcabamba, Peru; the Caucasus Mountains of the Soviet Union; and other places around the world.

Doctor-Patient Handbook

Discover the reversal process and healing crisis that Nature uses to rid the body of disease and restore well-being. Here is a fresh approach to wholistic health.

Slender Me Naturally

Dr. Jensen's answer to fad diets that don't work is a natural weight loss program that does. Developed over fifty-eight years of experience with overweight patients, this program is a healthful and effective way of losing unwanted weight.

Breathe Again Naturally

Get rid of asthma, allergies, bronchitis, hay fever, and other respiratory problems. Dr. Jensen discusses nutrition, herbs that work, food supplements, breathing exercises, attitude, and climate.

Arthritis, Rheumatism and Osteoporosis

Are you among the one in four Americans who suffers from arthritis, rheumatism, or osteoporosis? Would you like to know what to do about it? This book is for you.

Foods That Heal

This book presents the basic principles of Hippocrates, Dr. Rocine, and Dr. Jensen regarding the use of foods to help the body regain health. The author has also included a complete guide to the various fruits and vegetables we all need.

In Search of Shangri-La

Here is the very personal journal of Dr. Jensen's physical and spiritual travels through China into Tibet, and his reflections on his search for Shangri-La.

Love, Sex and Nutrition

Based on years of detailed study, this book explores the link between diet, sensuality, and relationships. This is an important and practical guide for people who wish to improve their sexuality safely and naturally.

For information regarding prices, write to:

Hidden Valley Health Ranch
Route 1 Box 52
Escondido, California 92025